More of
The World's Best Kept
Health Secret
REVEALED

Book 2

Leading
Wellness Doctors

The World's Best Kept Health Secret Revealed: Book 2

ISBN 0-9744857-1-3

1. Self-Help   I. The World's Best Kept Health Secret Revealed: Book 2
2. Health   I. The World's Best Kept Health Secret Revealed: Book 2

Book Layout/Design by Clark Kidman

Chiropractic Press books are available for distribution by emailing info@chiropracticpress.com or calling 715-868-1109.

Attention: Doctors of Chiropractic.
Are you a doctor of chiropractic who would like to become a published best selling author? If so, contact Chiropractic Press, Inc. at 715-868-1109 or email info@chiropracticpress.com for the free special report on how to become a published author.

Please Read This
Disclaimer Carefully

INDEMNITY.

You agree to defend, indemnify, and hold Chiropractic Press, Inc., its officers, directors, employees, agents, licensors, licensees, contributing authors/experts and suppliers, harmless from and against any claims, actions or demands, liabilities and settlements including without limitation, reasonable legal and accounting fees, resulting from, or alleged to result from, your violation of this Disclaimer.

GENERAL.

Chiropractic Press, Inc. is based in the United States of America. Chiropractic Press, Inc. and "Group" make no claims that the Book or the content is appropriate or may be used outside of the United States. Access to the content may not be legal by certain persons or in certain countries. If you access this Book or the content from outside the United States, you do so at your own risk and are responsible for compliance with the laws of your jurisdiction. The following provisions survive the expiration or termination of this Disclaimer for any reason whatsoever: Liability, Indemnity, Jurisdiction, and Complete Agreement.

JURISDICTION.

You expressly agree that exclusive jurisdiction for any dispute with Chiropractic Press, Inc. or "Group", or in any way relating to your use of this Book or content, resides in the courts of the State of Minnesota, United States of America, or it can be moved to a court and jurisdiction of Chiropractic Press, Inc.'s choice. You further agree and expressly consent to the exercise of personal jurisdiction in the courts of the State of Minnesota or a court and jurisdiction of Chiropractic Press, Inc.'s choice in connection with any such dispute including any claim involving Chiropractic Press, Inc. or its contributing experts, licensors, licensees, agents, affiliates, subsidiaries, employees, contractors, officers, directors and content providers.

The terms and conditions of this Disclaimer are governed by the internal substantive laws of the State of Minnesota, without respect to its conflict of law principles and can be moved to a court and jurisdication of Chiropractic Press, Inc's choice and approval. If any provision of this Disclaimer is found to be invalid by any court having competent jurisdiction, the invalidity of such provision shall not affect the validity of the remaining provisions of this Disclaimer, which shall remain in full force and effect. No waiver of any of this Disclaimer shall be deemed a further or continuing waiver of such term or condition or any other term or condition.

COMPLETE AGREEMENT.

This Disclaimer constitutes the entire agreement between you, Chiropractic Press, Inc. and "Group" with respect to the use of this Book and content.

If you do not wish to be bound by this disclaimer, please return this Book to the person who gave you this Book or the place you purchased it for a refund!

CONTENTS

꧁꧂

WHAT IS A DOCTOR OF CHIROPRACTIC?

Using the latest scientific and peer-reviewed research on subluxations, these leading wellness Doctors of Chiropractic explore how to provide you with new levels of energy, health and wellness. They show you ways to stop and reverse health challenges and make conscious choices that could transform your life and the lives of your loved ones. These doctors provide you information which could help you heal yourself and then, using what you have learned, help you heal your family.

Doctors of Chiropractic are trained to identify within the nervous system causes of poor health, illness and injuries. Without using drugs, invasive techniques or surgery, Doctors of Chiropractic help the body naturally reverse current health problems and prevent future ones. Each year, 30 million people choose this proven form of healthcare and wellnesscare.

What is a Doctor of Chiropractic? A Doctor of Chiropractic (D.C.) must go through schooling similar to medical doctors. With the same admission requirements as medical schools, chiropractic colleges require three to four years of undergraduate study with specific emphasis in science, biology, chemistry, physics and anatomy. Once accepted, chiropractic students complete *four to five years* of extensive study to achieve their Doctorate of Chiropractic. For chiropractic and medical students, the first two years of training are similar. Once past those years, chiropractic and medical students take separate routes. Medical students focus on pharmacology (drugs), critical care and surgery.

Chiropractic students focus on the central nervous system, methods of natural healing and the causes and effects of subluxation.

Prior to licensing as a Doctor of Chiropractic, the student must pass a multi-day, four-part National Board Examination. States also may require additional testing before granting state licensure. Each state has annual continuing education requirements Doctors of Chiropractic must complete to maintain their licenses.

Some patients have chosen Doctors of Chiropractic as primary physicians. This does not mean the chiropractor prescribes drugs. It means the patient goes to the chiropractor for most of his or her health concerns. The Primary Physician Chiropractor would either treat the patient with chiropractic techniques or natural healthcare or refer the patient to the appropriate healthcare provider.

CHAPTER ONE

HEALTH SECRET REVEALED

PART ONE

BRIDGING THE GAP

Dr. Allan A. Buratti, B.A., D.C., C.C.S.P

"The average physician treats the disease once it occurs. The better-than-average physician prevents the disease from coming back. The best physician prevents the disease from ever occurring." – Dr. Allan A. Buratti

The Wellness Revolution

We are at the forefront of a healthcare revolution. A new paradigm of healthcare designed to identify and reverse health problems before serious consequences arise.

More people are becoming aware of alternatives to drugs and surgeries. A number of people are choosing safer and more viable options before opting for medications or invasive surgeries. The chiropractic profession, with its focus on health and wellness, is uniquely suited to lead the Wellness Revolution into the 21st century.

What Is The Wellness Revolution?

The Wellness Revolution is choosing positive actions to keep you healthy and prevent illness. In contrast, crisis care is when you go to the doctor *after* you get sick.

Health problems don't just appear overnight. Given the right set of unfortunate circumstances, health problems and disease processes insidiously develop within our bodies. Whether it is the multiplication of malignant cells, a heart straining under the gradual blocking of the arteries, a malfunctioning pancreas or arthritis or osteoporosis, a series of events happens years before these conditions result in noticeable symptoms.

Although some people may have a genetic predisposition to certain health conditions, the vast majority of these conditions could be effectively managed if those negative influences were identified and eliminated before a crisis developed.

How Healthy Are You?

Your health status is the sum total of all the positive actions you take to preserve your well-being. This must be weighed against all the negative influences your body is bombarded with every day. There are many levels of health, ranging from 100 percent well-being to zero percent, or death. Think for a second about how you would define yourself along this scale. Do you realize it could be years after imbalances have occurred within your body before symptoms and diseases surface?

People with grapefruit-sized tumors, diabetes, coronary artery disease, thyroid disease and a variety of other conditions might have felt good for many years before they discovered their problems. These conditions are known to gradually build over time until symptoms are experienced.

In between the time of perfect health and disease could have been an opportunity to identify areas of dysfunction within the body and possibly reverse disease processes before they progressed into serious pathological conditions.

The Gap

As I see it, our current healthcare system has a huge division, or "gap," between perfect health and disease. On one side of the divide is wellness. On the other side is disease. What people do between these two extremes could determine the future of their health and their quality of lives.

Will you spend your golden years traveling and playing with your grandchildren? Or will you live a limited existence, unable to enjoy life to its fullest extent while grudgingly spending time and money shuffling from one doctor to the next?

What about those people who are in between? Stuck in the gap? You know who I'm talking about – individuals with chronic pain, fatigue, headaches, weakness or who just don't feel well. After months of being shuttled from one doctor to the next with endless arrays of tests, they may be told nothing is wrong. Where do these people fit in?

Let me ask you a question. If you came across a smoldering leaf in the woods, would you snuff it out before it started a forest fire? Or would you sit back and wait until an entire mountainside was engulfed in flames and then decide to put it out with a shot glass filled with water?

As absurd as this sounds, this is how a number of people view their health. They wait until their first stroke, heart attack or disc herniation before they feel the need to change their lifestyles or seek help from a wellnesscare professional.

Even then, many people think there is some magic pill or other quick fix that will return them to perfect health instantly. It is much easier to take measures to achieve a healthy state and maintain it, rather than wait for a life-threatening crisis to occur and try to reverse it.

Predictive Healthcare^{SM}

What if there was a way to predict future health problems? What if this knowledge enabled strategic measures to be taken to halt and reverse the dis-ease process? If you knew you might experience back problems or disc problems 10 years in the future, would you take heed and implement the necessary steps to prevent it?

In our office, we utilize treatment protocols designed to bridge the gap between chiropractic and traditional medicine through an integrated, multi-faceted approach to health. We call this approach Predictive Healthcare^{SM}. The goal of this system is to restore your body to optimum health through the identification and correction of structural and biochemical imbalances.

This is done by a careful analysis of the spine and body systems together with any necessary diagnostic tests of blood, urine, saliva and hair. These tests can provide a wealth of information to uncover subtle indications of impending areas of concern and lack of well-being. Once we discover the areas we need to correct, we customize a comprehensive treatment protocol. In a number of cases, the first step of treatment is the removal of subluxations.

What Are Subluxations?

As a Doctor of Chiropractic, it is my view one of the most overlooked negative influences on the human body is subluxation. A subluxation is a condition where a bone loses its proper position. This could interfere with the normal transmission of nerve impulses throughout the body.

A subluxation can be present in the spine, extremities, head or TMJ (jaw) and can go undetected for years before pain or a problem develops. In addition to possibly causing nerve interference, subluxations could lead to pain and an overall lack of well-being.

The network of nerves throughout the body originates from the spine. It is theorized a subluxation can impede the function of all the various organs, muscles and cells influenced by that particular level of the spine. When nerve interference is removed, the body's innate intelligence could have the ability to restore the body back to health.

Think of it this way. If a subluxation is located at the level of the spine adjacent to the nerves supplying information to the gallbladder, it could have the same effect on the gallbladder that a dimmer switch has on a light bulb. The affected organ may only function at 40 percent of normal, which possibly leads to digestive problems and gallbladder issues.

The more subluxations you have, the less "light" you may feel. The ability to optimally function or heal some health challenges may exist. A chiropractic adjustment removes the subluxation, and the "light" becomes brighter.

Having said all this, we must note that one or any combination of the following factors might cause subluxations:

1. **Physical stress** – injuries, poor posture, improper function of internal organs.
2. **Chemical stress** – nutritional deficiencies, food sensitivities, poor diet, chemicals.
3. **Emotional stress** – tension, fear, worry and anxiety from everyday life.
4. **Toxicity** – chemicals, pesticides, pollution, toxic metals overloading the body's ability to eliminate.

Just as a subluxation might cause interference to nerves that affect other areas of the body, problems in the body could lead to subluxations. In some cases, removal of subluxations and associated nerve interference is all that is needed to enable the body to restore itself back to health.

For more complicated cases, in addition to adjustments to remove subluxations, some of the following steps might be required for resolution of the problem:

- Remove nerve interference by correcting the subluxation
- Restore normal digestive function
- Restore normal elimination and bowel function
- Analyze proper nutritional needs
- Restore normal adrenal gland function
- Identify and eliminate offending foods
- Restore immune function
- Detoxify
- Restore hormone balance
- Adhere to proper diet and hydration

Same Problem, Different Solution

Two people can have the same condition or diagnosis, but the solutions may be completely different combinations of therapies. For example, in my experience as a doctor, someone with fibromyalgia might have subluxations in the neck, shoulder and jaw. Yet another person with this same condition may have subluxations to the mid-back. These could be perpetuated by improper digestion, which could lead to food allergies. Combine that with possible hormone imbalances, adrenal fatigue and various nutritional deficiencies.

It can be seen that when all the pieces of the puzzle are put together, the most effective, individualized treatment can be applied.

The Future Of Healthcare

I believe the future of 21st century healthcare should provide an integrated approach to achieving and maintaining wellness through the coordinated efforts of the chiropractic and medical professions. I see chiropractic care bridging the gap between health and dis-ease, and the medical profession providing crisis and emergency care. I believe the health of our nation would be improved and the quality of our lives would be greatly enhanced. I feel if a new paradigm of health included a strategic alliance between the chiropractic and medical fields, the patient would be armed with the best of both worlds.

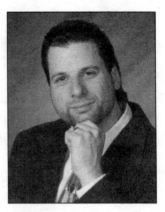

Dr. Allan A. Buratti, B.A., D.C., C.C.S.P.
Buratti Chiropractic Clinic
1882 Wayne Road
Chambersburg, Pennsylvania
(717) 261-0822

Dr. Buratti is Clinic Director of Buratti Chiropractic Center where he has maintained a thriving practice since 1991. His extensive knowledge and clinical background in so many specialized areas of healthcare enable him to provide an integrated approach to today's more complex health concerns, including anti-aging and wellness. In recognition of his accomplishments, Dr. Buratti received the prestigious honor of being selected as one of "America's Top Chiropractors" by the Consumer's Research Council of America.

Dr. Buratti received his Bachelor's Degree from Duquesne University and his Doctorate of Chiropractic degree from Palmer College of Chiropractic, where he graduated with honors.

His impressive postgraduate achievements include certification as a Chiropractic Sports Physician through Logan College of Chiropractic and the completion of several years of study in orthopedics, internal disorders and nutrition from National University of Health Sciences, Texas College of Chiropractic and Northwestern University of Health Sciences.

Realizing the need, Dr. Buratti established a new paradigm of wellness called Predictive Healthcare[SM], which decisively bridges the gap between traditional medicine and chiropractic. Through his life-long study in health and wellness, he has discovered specific approaches, techniques and strategies that significantly launch ordinary people to extraordinary health...youthful and energetic at most any age.

To schedule a private appointment or to arrange for Dr. Buratti to speak for your corporation or group, call (717) 261-0822.

PART TWO

CHIROPRACTORS ARE PART OF THE HEALTHCARE TEAM

Dr. Daniel Reida, D.C.

"Your Daddy's a bone crusher."
"Your Daddy's a witch doctor."
"Your Daddy's not a real doctor."
"Your Daddy's a quack."

Yes, those were common phrases thrown my way growing up as the son of a chiropractor in the 1960s. In the 1970s, when I became a practicing chiropractor, my patients were commonly told by their medical doctors, "If you ever go back to him, don't ever come back to me."

Of course, the medical doctors didn't know *me* at all, other than the fact I was a chiropractor.

Thirty or forty years ago, traditional medicine was massively accepted and rarely questioned. Chiropractic was constantly questioned and almost off the radar screen in healthcare. Back then, the public perception of medical doctors had them up on pedestals while Doctors of Chiropractic were deemed second-class citizens.

Fast forward to 2004. Oh my goodness, how things have changed.

Medicine is being challenged at all levels and some medical

doctors are paying over $100,000 a year for malpractice insurance. Chiropractic is among the most overwhelmingly popular complementary and alternative medicines (CAM) and we pay about $2,500 per year for our malpractice insurance.

The healthcare consumer has become much more sophisticated, informed and demanding. The healthcare consumer now can choose care through medicine, chiropractic, massage therapy, acupuncture, naturopathy, Reiki energy healing, nutritionists, herbalists and more.

According to a survey conducted by the National Center for Complementary and Alternative Medicine, the United States public spent an estimated $36 billion to $47 billion on Complementary and Alternative Medicine in 1997. Of this amount, between $12 billion and $20 billion was paid out-of-pocket for the services of professional Complementary and Alternative Medicine (CAM) healthcare providers, such as Doctors of Chiropractic. People spent more out-of-pocket with CAM healthcare providers and doctors than for medical doctor services.

I believe these patients are much more health-conscious and well-informed. More people now utilize the Internet to answer their healthcare questions than ask their medical doctors

The Massachusetts Chiropractic Society (Masschiro.org) recently hired a firm called Titanium, Inc. from North Hampton, Massachusetts to survey existing chiropractic patients, former patients and people who have never utilized chiropractic. The purpose was to develop a picture of how chiropractic is viewed and utilized.

The data is quite interesting:

- Currently, approximately 10 percent of the public uses chiropractic on a regular basis.
- Another 10 percent to 20 percent of the public is interested and leaning towards using chiropractic care (as many as 77 million people), but they don't know enough about it to make an informed decision.

- More than 70 percent of chiropractic patients specified back and neck problems as their health problems for which they sought chiropractic care.

This opinion is supported by several research findings:
- Chiropractic is clinically proven to be an effective treatment for lower back pain.
- More than 11.7 million Americans are significantly impaired and 2.6 million are permanently disabled by back pain.
- Fifty percent of working age people experience back symptoms each year.
- Back symptoms are the most common cause of disability for people under 45 years old.
- Low back problems are the second most common symptomatic reason for visits to physicians.

Chiropractors are now accurately viewed as being part of patients' healthcare teams. Patients no longer rely on any one doctor. They choose a medical doctor, Doctor of Chiropractic, a massage therapist, a nutritionist and so on.

According to a national survey entitled *Perceptions About Complementary Therapies Relative to Conventional Therapies Among Adults Who Use Both*, 79 percent of respondents believe using both conventional and alternative therapies are superior to either one alone. It also revealed that patient confidence in CAM providers was the same as confidence in medical providers.

Chiropractors, by training and licensing standards, are well equipped to diagnose and treat or to diagnose and refer to other appropriate providers.

Here is an interesting piece of data uncovered in our survey and research. With respect to 53 primary care functions found to occur daily in medical offices, chiropractors are capable of making diagnoses in 92 percent of these activities and making therapeutic contributions in more than 50 percent of them.

In the past few months in my practice, I have helped hundreds of patients with back problems of many origins including work injuries, auto accident injuries, slip and fall injuries, yard work injuries and other common injuries.

I've also had cases during that time which demonstrate the importance of having a Doctor of Chiropractic on your healthcare team.

A 63-year-old male patient of mine developed severe low back and leg pains following a prostate surgery. He had an MRI of his low back followed by Facet injections by a medical doctor and found no relief.

The pain was so bad I made house calls (yes, I still make house calls) to the patient's house 10 days in a row. He couldn't get out of his bed for the first five days due to the back pain. When the patient could stand and walk, I referred him back to his neurosurgeon. The neurosurgeon referred him for physical therapy.

The problem worsened with physical therapy. On a Tuesday evening, I ordered another MRI. At 9:30 a.m. Wednesday, the Chief of Radiology called me to report the patient had osteomyelitis, a potentially life-threatening infection of the bone of his spine. I referred him to the hospital where other specialists took over. He has now recovered.

Billy, a 58-year-old male patient of mine, called me at my home over a holiday weekend on May 26, 2003 to receive emergency treatment for low back pain. It seemed similar to a problem he had a year ago which I had treated. On May 27, 2003, he returned still in terrible pain. He reported a fever and had already gone to his medical doctor that morning.

I asked if the medical doctor had ordered blood and urine tests to rule out kidney infection. Billy said yes and all was okay. Probing further, I asked if he had any recent puncture wounds or cuts. He said no but that he had had a deer tick bite. It resulted in an inflammatory reaction in December. Six days after the bite, he had a Lyme's disease test that was negative. I told Billy, Lyme's disease tests will often test negative for one month after the bite. I referred Billy for a Lyme's disease test as well as a complete blood count and an arthritis profile.

On the morning of Wednesday, May 28, 2003, Billy returned still having acute low back pain and fever. He had not gone for the blood tests. Now his pain was across the low back in the kidney area. I insisted he go directly to the blood lab and be tested for Lyme's disease as well as a kidney profile and CBC (complete blood count). His wife Barbara was with him because he couldn't drive with the immense pain. Barbara drove him to the lab where the tests were completed.

About 4:15 p.m. that same Wednesday afternoon, the lab called me to report some serious abnormal test results. I immediately called Billy and Barbara to report the findings, directing them to go immediately to their medical doctor. They weren't home. I left a message on their machine.

About 15 minutes later, Barbara returned my call. I told her my concerns and to take Billy directly to their medical doctor. At 5:30 p.m., Barbara called to let me know she had contacted their medical doctor who said to go to the emergency room at Cape Cod Hospital. The next morning, Barbara called me with an update that Billy was going for an MRI of the low back.

At 3:15 p.m. Barbara phoned saying the results of the MRI had shown possible bone cancer or osteomyelitis, which is a potentially life-threatening infection of the bone of the spine. Billy was admitted to Brigham and Women's Hospital with aggressive osteomyelitis. Billy was told if he had waited just eight hours longer, he could have died.

Billy and Barbara are incredibly thankful for my thoroughness and fast action, which saved his life. It was a combination of long, extensive training, years of experience as a doctor, persistence and human compassion that helped me identify and know the course of action to resolve this health situation. This shows the importance of having a Doctor of Chiropractic on your healthcare team.

Jillian, a delightful 3-year-old girl, was brought in by her mother, Mona, for a most unusual problem — chronic night terrors. Mona described the problem to me. Over a year ago, Jillian had had four front teeth removed because of damage from "bottle rot." The surgery had no apparent complications until Jillian went to sleep that night, and every night since.

Jillian's mother said Jillian would sleep the first two hours. Then, Jillian would awaken hysterically crying and screaming every hour for the rest of the night. This continued night after night for a year. Mona said the pediatrician had no explanation except, "Jillian must be going through a phase."

Mona was certainly "going through a phase" by the time one of her friends suggested chiropractic care, and she arrived in my office.

After a thorough history and examination, I detected vertebral subluxations in Jillian's spine. Vertebral subluxations happen when spinal bones become misaligned or a little out of normal position. This can affect the spinal nerves. Spinal nerves carry messages to and from the brain and all parts of the body. Chiropractors know any interference in the nervous system could affect body functions.

Chiropractors are extensively trained to know nerve impulses flow from the brain down the spinal cord, out the spinal nerves between the vertebrae to all parts of the body. The nerve impulses return through similar pathways to the brain. This is called the Loop System. If this Loop System is over-stimulated or under-stimulated from subluxation problems, the body could malfunction.

I didn't know for sure if correcting Jillian's subluxations would stop her night terrors, but I told Mom I would take Jillian on a trial basis for six weeks. I recommended one adjustment per week for the six weeks. If Jillian was improving, we would continue.

I gave Jillian her first adjustment and saw her a week later. Mom said Jillian's sleeping and screaming was even worse during that first week. I was encouraged because I knew we had made a change that seemed related to her problems.

I adjusted her again. Mom and Jillian returned. Jillian had slept through one whole night. Yahoo! During week three, Jillian slept through four nights in a row.

Wow, Jillian's life has changed so much for the better. Jillian's Mom, Mona, can sleep again. Jillian's pediatrician who wrote her prescription for chiropractic care is surprised and pleased.

After 33 years of practice, I continue to marvel at the wide varieties of problems we help. It is so good to work as a team.

These examples demonstrate the many ways Doctors of Chiropractic can help patients. Even if we can't treat the exact problem, we can refer people to the doctors who can because we are part of the patient's healthcare team.

Chiropractors have excellent working relationships with the blood labs, the radiology departments, the MRI centers, physical therapy departments and other diagnostic facilities.

Doctors of Chiropractic can pick up the phone and refer our patients to many different specialists such as neurologists, orthopedic surgeons, neurosurgeons, physical therapists or back to primary care physicians. Often, we continue to co-treat the patient while the other doctor treats the patient's other complaints.

Chiropractors are known for their willingness to take the time to listen to patients, to view overall health and to take the time to explain health problems with more natural perspectives. Patients want to know their options with healthcare. That's why they choose to have Doctors of Chiropractic on their healthcare teams.

Chiropractic is safe, comfortable and is cost-effective. Chiropractic is the best care for most back and neck problems with the highest patient satisfaction.

For the patient's benefit, we're team players on the healthcare team.

Dr. Dan Reida, D.C.
Practicing Family Chiropractor
President, Cape Cod Chiropractic Society
Board of Director, Massachusetts
Chiropractic Society
Past-President, The International
Chiropractic Knights of the Roundtable

Bass River Healthcare Associates, Inc.
833 Main Street – Route 28
South Yarmouth, Massachusetts 02664-5240
(508)394-1353
neuraxis@aol.com
www.bassriverhealthcare.com

In addition to full time practice since 1972, Dr. Dan Reida is president of the Cape Cod Chiropractic Society and Board of Director of the Massachusetts Chiropractic Society. Dr. Reida is also a member of, and past president of, one of the most prestigious chiropractic organizations, The International Chiropractic Knights of the Roundtable.

Dr. Reida is a sought-after speaker who has lectured nationally and internationally since 1984 to chiropractic colleagues and the public. He has taught at seminars for professional advancement and at Palmer College of Chiropractic for continuing education programs. Dr. Reida is credentialed by The American Board of Independent Medical Examiners as an Independent Chiropractic Examiner.

Besides professional success, Dr. Reida has been a dedicated father and taught Fatherhood Seminars and was awarded Big Brother of the Year in 1996 for his extensive work for the Big Brother/Big Sister program. Dr. Reida has also been a serious athlete having run over 22,000 miles and completed seven triathlons including one of Ironman distance. In 2002, Dr. Reida completed one of his lifetime goals of riding almost 2,000 miles across Alaska to the Arctic Circle and back with his 21-year-old son Austin. They rode one cylinder dual sport motorcycles across miles of dirt and mud.

To schedule a private appointment with Dr. Reida or to arrange for Dr. Reida to speak to your corporation or group, call (508)394-1353.

PART THREE

Chiropractic Is Only A Secret To Those Who Haven't Discovered It Yet

❧

Dr. Alex Kassalias, D.C.

Each year many people are enjoying the most popular, natural, drug-free health care system in the world.

For those of you who are still in search of true health and wellness, I would like my chapter to serve as an instrument to clear up misinformation. I encounter people who have never experienced chiropractic. They like to tell me what they think chiropractic treatments are like. I usually hear them say, "I'll call you if my back hurts."

Some are surprised when I tell them chiropractic is used to treat more than just back pain. This stuns them! In my practice people of all ages learn chiropractic can help them function closer to their physical and emotional best, and may even help them recover faster from a number of illnesses and disabilities. Some even realize they have less need for drugs and sometimes no longer require surgery! I believe chiropractic patients enjoy life more fully with less stress and more energy.

What Is Chiropractic?

Chiropractic is a system of health care that releases serious stress from your body by relieving misalignments of your spine called subluxations. A subluxation could affect your nerves, muscles, bones, internal organs, brain function, posture and overall health.

How Do We Get Subluxations?

Subluxations occur when misaligned spinal bones, called vertebra, put pressure on the spinal nerves that come out from between each of the vertebra. The pressure on these nerves interferes with normal nerve signals traveling to various parts of the body.

Subluxations can be caused by many types of stress. These can include poor posture, accidents, sitting in the same position in the car or in front of a computer, sports and even emotional and chemical stress. People can have subluxations in their bodies caused by birth or childhood falls. Unless they have a chiropractic checkup and subsequent treatment, these long-standing subluxations could cause problems throughout their entire lives.

So the secret is out. Chiropractic, in my opinion, is not a belief, religion or a theory. It is a healing art, science and vitalistic philosophy. Discoveries and developments in chiropractic have spanned more than 100 years of exact research and careful testing.

What Is Wellness?

To explain wellness, let's look at physiology – how your body works. A human body is made up of billions of tiny packets of life called cells. Cells are constantly engaging with each other – vibrating, chemically communicating with each other as energies organize them from a formless mass into a living body.

Cells organize to form tissues. Tissues form organs. Organs evolve into systems such as your digestive system or circulatory system, etc. When all systems are working in a harmonious, coordinated fashion, they create a healthy, self-regulating living body.

What then makes all these structures come "alive" as they

engage each other and chemically communicate to work together? A corpse has all of the same parts as a living body, but it is not alive. Missing is the life energy of the body, also called innate intelligence. This energy directs chemical reactions and nerve signals and communicates to the whole body by sending information through your nervous system. Your nervous system includes the brain, spinal cord and billions of nerve fibers that communicate with every cell.

This flow of energy is necessary to organize the activities the body performs every second. If the nervous system is blocked or stressed, this fantastic communication system could suffer from interference. This interference could cause disease or more aptly "dis-ease." Simply put, the parts aren't able to work in harmony.

You see, how human bodies work is not merely a chiropractic point of view, a belief or some sort of religion. This is the science of living things. This is why a body free of interference or subluxation is able to function properly.

How Does Chiropractic Work?

The adjustment is a method chiropractors use to help correct vertebral subluxations. Doctors of Chiropractic are the only healthcare professionals specifically trained to locate, analyze and correct subluxations. In fact, many state licensing boards require completion of a four-year chiropractic college course following at least two years of undergraduate education, with some states requiring a bachelor's degree before chiropractic training and/or before licensure.

Who Should Visit A Chiropractor?

I had a medical doctor ask me this question. He was surprised when I proclaimed, "Everybody!" I believe every person should have his or her spine checked for subluxations. Correcting subluxations might help achieve wellness.

I've been telling this to countless people over the ten years I have been in practice. I have many contacts and relationships with the medical doctors, nurses and other health care professionals in my community. Some refer their patients to me for chiropractic care to complement their own care. Some health care professionals and their families are even my patients. They say it best.

Dr. Ivet E. Hudson, M.D., Family Medicine says, "In medical practice I diagnose and treat various symptoms, complaints and illnesses. I have personally worked with Dr. Kassalias for some time now. His chiropractic practice is different than traditional medicine because it is concerned with improving wellness. Chiropractic is not just for neck problems and back pain, but optimizing the nervous system and pathways, which control every function in the body. This is why spinal misalignments (subluxations) can be detrimental to one's health."

From Dr. Ron Gardener, M.D., Radiologist, "Dr. Kassalias is well versed in the analysis and diagnosis of X-ray study. Dr. Kassalias and I have had many clinical conversations over the years on X-ray findings and patient protocols. In my medical specialty, I literally will read over a thousand X-rays per month, which takes its toll on my own posture and spinal function. I've seen the changes that Dr. Kassalias has made by reviewing X-rays, before and after chiropractic adjustments, and how he has restored the natural posture and curves in the spine. I decided to be one of his chiropractic patients."

A note from Greenville High School Nurse Gay Hawkins states, "I have been a nurse for twenty-nine years. I am writing this to let you know how misinformed I was about chiropractic care.

A teacher where I work was talking about how much Dr. Kassalias helped her. I personally had excruciating pain down my left leg. I went to the office and was very impressed with how comprehensive his examination was. He told me up front that if there was something he could not help me with, he would refer me to a specialist who could. He found areas in my spinal column with serious nerve blockages. The treatments I received were very gentle and specific. I couldn't believe the relief I experienced when conventional medicine failed. My energy levels are through the roof, and I did not get a cold all winter. I think all high school students should have a chiropractic check-up."

Dorothy Ross, RN wrote, "I saw my Internist and GYN professional and had no relief of symptoms. Searching for a reason for my problems, I decided to try something different. I found Dr. Kassalias and chiropractic care. Bless you and thank you, Dr. Kassalias, for my relief."

Wendy Rampey, MHS and Physical Therapist says, "Until I pursued chiropractic care for myself, I never fully realized its role in family wellness. From personal experience, I see (what) benefits chiropractic care has to offer and often recommend chiropractic care to my patients. Using an interdisciplinary approach to care can be quite beneficial. In physical therapy, the musculoskeletal system's flexibility, strength and stability are assessed and treated with therapeutic exercise and mobilizations to improve functional status. Chiropractic care, however, includes assessing dysfunction and mal-alignment in the spinal column, which may inevitably affect nervous system integrity and function. By using a holistic approach, physical therapy used in conjunction with chiropractic care can reduce symptoms, improve function and prevent unnecessary surgical interventions."

Sherilyn D. Breazeale, Licensed Veterinary Technician says, "I have been in the veterinary field since 1986. While volunteering time to work with abandoned and abused animal cases, I have assisted in the treatment and operations on countless animals, from minor to very severe and complicated procedures. I have witnessed situations when injured dogs and cats or, at times, post surgical animals, have not recovered to their full potential because of a vertebral misalignment in the spine. This misalignment was not allowing proper nerve supply to the animal's extremities or vital organs. This is common in animals hit by cars that suffer pelvic and other bone injuries. This problem results in lameness and bodily dysfunction. I have called on my friend, Dr. Alex Kassalias, to perform specific adjustments to the spinal misalignments, which opened up nerve supply. This almost always proves success to the animal's condition within days. One should never underestimate the power of the God-given healing ability in all living things."

Yes, it is true! Chiropractors can even take certification classes in animal-adjusting techniques. Dogs and cats, or any creature with spinal misalignments, could actually experience wellness with chiropractic care!

I am trained in a number of modern, effective and gentle techniques through my hundreds of hours of post-graduate studies. Every patient is different. I am careful to choose techniques that most benefit their particular situations. This wide range of care includes techniques gentle enough for infants, seniors and post-surgical patients, yet effective enough to treat active teens, hardworking adults and injured athletes. I believe through chiropractic care, everyone can benefit and achieve wellness.

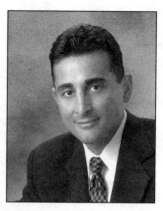

Dr. Alex Kassalias, D.C.
Family Chiropractor
701 Congaree Road
Greenville, South Carolina 29607
(864) 297-3000

At the young age of 15, Dr. Alex Kassalias discovered the benefits of chiropractic. When Alex injured his back while training for a major high school weight lifting competition, the team coach recommended a local chiropractor to speed Alex's recovery. The first adjustment introduced his body to its own healing ability. The benefits chiropractic care offered Alex led to his advancement in State and National Level Power Lifting and Body Building Championships. With trophies won, he pursued a much more powerful calling, becoming a chiropractor. Dr. Kassalias now has a family practice in Greenville, South Carolina where every day he helps others reach their true life potential.

To schedule a private appointment with Dr. Kassalias or to arrange for Dr. Kassalias to speak to your corporation or group, call (864) 297-3000.

PART FOUR

HOW TO CHOOSE WELLNESS

❧

Dr. Robert Bocknek, D.C.

The central nervous system is important to your overall wellness. To understand the importance of the central nervous system you have to go all the way back to the beginning.

When an egg is fertilized, cells begin to divide into a small circular mass with a long, thin cord ascending from this mass. This is the brain and spinal cord, which are the first organs to develop in the womb. Little branches of nerves begin to grow from the spinal cord equally on both sides of the cord. The combination of your brain, spinal cord and nerves becomes your central nervous system. Right from the beginning, you can see how important the central nervous system is to the human body — it's the first thing to develop!

Next, at the end of each nerve grows a bud. The first bud is your heart, then your liver, your kidneys and your spleen. This continues until all your organs are formed. Your organs grow out of your nervous system.

Protection For Your Nervous System

Once the organs are formed, the body begins to build protection for your central nervous system by growing a skull around the brain.

Next, bones called vertebrae grow around the spinal cord to protect it. The vertebrae are joints with holes on each side so the nerves can run through the bones to the organs and be protected at the same time. This is your spinal column. The central nervous system is the pathway for signals to travel from the brain and to tell the cells what to do next.

The spinal column was created to be flexible. While the body is moving, messages travel from the brain, down the spinal cord, through the nerves and out to the organs, muscles and cells of the body and then back to the brain without interruption. Electrical impulses flowing over a healthy central nervous system free of interference can be a critical factor in the body's survival.

To help prevent message interruption over this critical pathway, the body even creates a backup system to make sure messages get through.

This system is called a nerve plexus. There are four plexuses – the cervical plexus, the lumbar plexus, the sacral plexus and the brachial plexus. Nerves within each plexus leave the spine, separate and splice again before connecting to a particular area. If there is an interruption in the nerve that goes to an organ, for instance, the signal may be rerouted through a different nerve. There are multiple plexuses in the neck region and the lower back. Located at critical places, the plexuses attempt to make sure a signal is able to get through, even if it is not a full signal.

Our nervous system was created to make sure the electrical signals traveling from the brain through the spinal cord have every chance to get where each signal needs to be in the body.

Aging Could Affect Your Nervous System

As we grow older, we could disrupt the critical flow of energy over this all-important system. We sit hunched over our school desks. We might not eat, stretch or exercise properly. Playing football, skiing, riding horses, falling off bikes or car accidents could also affect the body's ability to send and receive these vital electrical messages. Can you see how your spinal column could get knocked and rocked out of place?

Poor nutrition, bumps and jarring could misalign your spine causing a shift or twist in your spine's natural alignment. This misalignment, called subluxation, could create disruptions to your body's information superhighway – the central nervous system.

Not all of our nerves perceive pain. You may not "feel" a health problem. Have you ever gone to a dentist and been told you had a cavity, even though you never felt any pain? Would you tell the dentist, "I have no pain, so I am not going to fix the cavity?"

Seemingly healthy people have heart attacks even though they may have felt fine before the attacks. Were they fine the day before the heart attack?

Again, only a small portion of the nervous system perceives pain. If this part of the nervous system isn't affected, you may not feel pain. Other tracts of the sensory nerves of the nervous system respond to hot, cold or vibration. What does this mean? Only about 10 percent of our nerves respond to pain.

Feeling Your Best

Our bodies contain a system to maintain wellness. The choices one makes on a daily basis either brings health to or breaks down our bodies. We spend a lifetime undermining our health with poor eating habits, poor posture, lack of exercise and spinal adjustments. Then we may wonder why we are not feeling our best.

It takes only a small amount of pressure to interrupt a signal to and from the brain. Nerve interference between the brain and an organ could cause distorted messages.

For example, let's say a message leaves an empty stomach and is distorted on its way to the brain. The distorted version of the message tells the brain the stomach is full. The brain's response might be to signal the stomach to produce stomach acid to help digest food. But because the message was distorted and the stomach is actually empty, the person may suffer from a bout of heartburn although the brain thought it responded to the message appropriately.

I believe true wellness is achieved when the brain receives accurate information from the body. A properly functioning nervous system, free of interference caused by subluxations, could deliver 100 percent of the information 100 percent of the time.

I believe removing subluxations is a big part of achieving wellness. Chiropractic adjustments could be critical to helping the body's nervous system exchange accurate information. But what happens if you do not take the time to maintain your nervous system?

The brain wants to protect the nerves at all cost. To protect the nerves running through the joints of your spine, the brain may send a message to the muscles around the nerves, causing them to stiffen.

But the brain soon realizes it takes a lot of energy to keep the muscles tense. It needs to find a more efficient way of protecting its nerves. Where the muscles have stiffened the joints, it covers the spine in layers of calcium. After a couple of years you'll have new bone growing over the joint to protect the nerve. Sounds good, doesn't it? Well, it's not. That new bone growth is spondylitis, a form of arthritis — a painful, debilitating disease. Arthritis is not a strange problem only for seniors. It could be an end result of untreated subluxations and the resultant stiff joints.

A New Way Of Thinking

Our grandparents might have thought it normal to wear dentures as they aged. Now we see far fewer cavities and more people with great teeth. Could this be because it now seems normal to brush, floss and get regular dental check ups?

What if our children were to get regular spinal checkups from a chiropractor? What if they were to learn early on how to take care of their spines and the benefits good spinal hygiene could have for their health? Can you imagine as that happens how the health of the world would improve? It could be huge!

Each day we have choices. We could do something that could further breakdown the body. Or we could do something that will put us one step closer to wellness. Implementing regular chiropractic adjustments, healthy diet, regular exercise and stretching in our daily choices are the first steps I recommend to overall wellness.

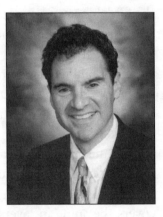

Dr. Robert Bocknek, D.C.
Bocknek Family Chiropractic
320 E. Maple Avenue, Suite C
Vienna, Virginia 22180
(703) 242-3533
DrBocknek@yahoo.com

Dr. Robert Bocknek, D.C. is the Best Selling Author of *The World's Best Kept Health Secret Revealed*. In addition, Dr. Bocknek is a Doctor of Chiropractic providing care to the Fairfax County, Northern Virginia area. Through his 19 year chiropractic career, he has discovered specific systems, behaviors and strategies that significantly launch ordinary people to extraordinary youthfulness and energetic health at most any age.

Dr. Bocknek has led thousands of individuals and families in the quest for maximum growth and wellness. His combination chiropractic, exercise, diet and nutrition workshops have been huge successes for health conscious and health unconscious alike. Dr. Bocknek's easy to follow steps are a must for anyone trying to bring vibrant health and joy back to his or her life.

As a speaker, Dr. Bocknek delivers a dynamic and inspirational program revealing the surprising and little-known systems of those who have achieved optimal health and wellness. Dr. Bocknek will give you the step-by-step action plan to super-charge your ability to overcome the negative results of stress and poor health.

Dr. Bocknek is a sought-after expert, speaker and media guest. He has spoken to corporations and business groups from Virginia to Taipei,

Taiwan. Dr. Bocknek captivates audiences through his keynotes and trainings on *The World's Best Kept Health Secret Revealed*. His new radio health show, *The World's Best Kept Health Secret Revealed*, can be heard in the Washington metro area.

Dr. Bocknek's proven health system has been so well accepted that his book has sold over 25,000 copies!

To schedule a private appointment with Dr. Bocknek or to arrange for Dr. Bocknek to speak to your corporation or group, call (703) 242-3533.

PART FIVE

HEALTH LOST

❦

Dr. Robert R. Mariner, B.S., D.C.

Pain. Sickness. Disease. Where do they come from? In varying stages and degrees, they all come from " health lost."

So why do we wait until we *lose* our health before we start to get concerned about it? Why do we wait until a sign or symptom arises before we decide to do something about it?

Let me answer that one for you. Human nature.

It also has to do with the way we were brought up. After all, we only know what we've been taught.

How Do We Get Health Back?

Does health come from prescriptive drugs? Does health come from surgery? Does health really come from *anything* outside of the body?

I believe health comes from our God-given "innate intelligence."

I view innate intelligence as a life force working through our nervous system. Our nervous system controls and coordinates all functions within the body. Interference could hamper its effectiveness.

I believe this innate intelligence uses the brain, spinal cord and nerves to orchestrate a symphony of communicative nerve impulses. These mental impulses *give life* to every cell of the body every second, every minute, every hour of every day.

The brain is the command center, the powerhouse and the central processing unit. It sends out thousands of mental impulse instructions while simultaneously receiving countless responses — all within seconds!

Wow! What computer can do all this?

Nerve impulses, generated from conscious and unconscious thoughts, stream from the brain to the spinal cord. They continue out the nerve roots exiting the different levels of the spine reaching each and every tissue of the body.

Cells, tissues and organs are all receiving instructions while sending messages back and forth through the conduit of electrical nerve wires.

Like little cars traveling on a freeway, billions of nerve impulses flow. They light up the way as they are traveling from home to work and then work to home. From the brain to the cell and the cell to brain.

This happens harmoniously as long as there is no interference. No jams clogging the nerve freeways. No accidents to slow down the flow of nerve traffic.

Chiropractors refer to these interferences, these accidents, these clogs in nerve flow as vertebral subluxations. Vertebral subluxations are abnormal positioning or motioning of the spinal vertebrae. They could lead to nerve interference.

Your heart. Your lungs. Your stomach. Your intestines. Your liver. Your kidneys. Everything in your body has a nerve supply. Subluxation could interfere with it.

These subluxations could initiate other soft tissue problems. These problems are associated more with the mechanics of the body. Specifically, this includes the muscles, tendons, ligaments and cartilage.

Subluxations could contribute in a huge way to a diminishing and downward spiraling of health.

What Could Cause Subluxations?

Car accidents. Falls. Bad sleeping positions. Poor posture. Environmental pollution. Mental and emotional pollution.

Sports injuries. Riding all day in a car. Sitting all day at work. Standing in one position for a long time. Bad pillows. Wrong mattresses. Unsupportive shoes.

What else?

Poor biomechanics. Gardening for a long period of time. Bending over the bed while making it. Working behind a computer too long. Operating a computer mouse incorrectly. The birthing process.

Subluxations can also be caused by any one-sided body activity repeated over time. Examples of this include sitting on a thick wallet in your back pocket or wearing a shoulder purse on the same side all the time.

These one-sided activities could lead to an imbalance within the body. This imbalance could lead to furthering subluxations. A snowballing effect could be set into motion, paving the way for an opportunistic crisis to occur.

My one word description for the cause of subluxations is………*stress!*

Anything that stresses our bodies, whether it is a physical, chemical, mental or emotional stressor, could cause subluxations to build up.

Then…wham! You might experience pain, sickness or dis-ease.

The next question is very logical, "Who doesn't have stress?"

That's right! Everyone on God's green earth has stress! It could be stress of various types and degrees from mild to severe.

The next logical question is this, "If everyone has some degree of stress, doesn't *everyone* have some degree of subluxation?"

Since everyone could have the potential for some degree of subluxation, should everybody see a chiropractor?

I believe an important part of caring for health is to reduce subluxation stress, pressure and misalignment. This could allow the body to heal itself. It might prevent future problems. I include it in my health regimen with the goal of increasing health and wellness.

I also believe it is important for people to have their family members checked for subluxations. Your spouse. Your children. Your friends. *Everybody!*

I see pain, numbness, tingling, headaches and decreased range of motion as *alarms* going off in the body. It's innate intelligence trying to warn of a potentially neglected condition that could be causing damage.

If you set your alarm clock to go off in the morning at six and you keep hitting the snooze button, you're going to awaken late.

Similarly, if the pain alarm in your body goes off, and you ignore it or take a pain remedy to cover it up, you're hitting the "snooze button" without treating the *cause* of the alarm. You're masking the symptom. You're killing the messenger without acting on the message.

If the "check engine" light goes on in your car, would you cover it with a piece of masking tape so you couldn't see it and think, "There! That'll fix it!"

Yet, I believe that is precisely what people do when they cover up a problem with pain medication.

If symptoms are continually masked with medications, could it be that a problem is being covered up that may some day, literally, cover you up before your time?

I feel pain *signals* are trying to tell you things have been let go for too long. I believe these signals are trying to tell you, in a belated way, to get the problem fixed! I feel your chiropractor is a good resource.

Better yet, visit a chiropractor before you even develop the problem!

Remember, each individual vertebra of your spine works like a circuit breaker does in your house, with one exception.

If a circuit breaker in your house kicks, you lose *all* electricity to that area. If a vertebral circuit breaker kicks (subluxates), you may only lose *part* of the electrical flow through that nerve.

If it subluxates mildly, you may not have any pain or dysfunction until it subluxates further.

If you have a bad electrical connection going to a light bulb, the light bulb gets dim or it flickers. The same thing could happen if you have a vertebral subluxation pinching or choking a nerve root. The organ, tissue or gland supplied by the electrical nerve root, flickers with pain and dims with dysfunction.

Your spine could become out of alignment and out of balance, just like the front end of your car. When the front end of your car is out of alignment and out of balance, you take it to an auto mechanic to be straightened. This prevents your car from pulling to one side of the road. The mechanic will also balance the tires on the right and left so the car rides smoother.

I see the human vehicle in much the same way. Only it's the "back end" that gets out of alignment and out of balance. This time, you take your human vehicle to a human body mechanic who straightens out the back end and balances you right and left. Then, your ride could be healthier and smoother.

If you've ever had electrical problems with your car, then you know how troublesome they can be and the crazy things that can go wrong.

I make the same comparison with electrical or nerve problems with the human vehicle.

What kind of analogy can be made of a compressed, choked or pinched nerve?

Well, it's a lot like the feeling you get if you put your tongue between your teeth and then bite down on it. Or it's like walking around with a pebble in your shoe all the time.

Let me paint you another picture of what a pinched nerve is like.

Take a rubber band and wrap it around the end of your index finger. If you do this, you'd discover you're beginning to feel the blood and nerve supply being cut off at the end of your finger.

Now, you can treat the finger a lot of different ways.

You can take an aspirin or a prescription drug of some type, but would that solve the problem? Would exercising the end of your finger solve the problem? Would putting electrical therapy or ultrasound on the end of your finger solve the problem?

No. None of these things would solve the problem.

How about surgery? Surgically removing the end of the finger might solve the problem, but it certainly would *create* other problems!

Sounds *crazy*, doesn't it? But that's exactly what happens with a lot of people.

The obvious answer is to adjust the rubber band, loosening it up until all the pressure is removed from the nerve in the finger. Innate intelligence, on its own, then *heals* the finger!

That's exactly what could happen when a chiropractor adjusts the spine to relieve the pressure on a pinched nerve.

Now don't get me wrong. One adjustment doesn't remove all the nerve interference. Often it takes repeated adjustments before innate intelligence could take over in the healing department.

The results of your care could occur in a similar fashion to that of a brick foundation when building a house.

The first row of bricks, or the first adjustment, may not look like much. It is a start. Each row of bricks or adjustments that follows depends on the one made before it.

Sooner or later, depending on how many bricks or adjustments need to be made, you'll see and feel results!

Subluxations can stress muscles causing them to knot up, too, just like a rope can be knotted. Adjustments help get the knots out.

But if you don't get adjusted those knots could become chronic and fibrous. It's a lot like the gristle you find in a piece of steak.

When you go to a chiropractor for the first time, x-rays will likely be taken. X-rays serve as a "blueprint" for the chiropractor to help him or her visualize where the spine needs to be adjusted.

After analyzing the X-ray blueprints, a course of treatment is set and adjusting can begin.

The questions going through your mind at this point may be, "What is it like to be adjusted? Does it hurt? Is it safe? Will I have to keep coming back forever?"

Let's address some of these questions.

When you are adjusted, there is often a popping sound. This is not "bone crunching." It is the release of nitrogenous joint gases. When you are adjusted, the chiropractor is releasing misalignment, stress and subluxation pressure. This pressure release is stress relief!

Chiropractic adjustments don't usually hurt. In fact, most patients say it feels good to be adjusted. But, if you have any discomfort, just let your chiropractor know about it so less adjusting energy can be used on your next visit.

I believe chiropractic care is just about the safest thing in healthcare. No one has ever been paralyzed or died from any adjustments that I've ever given! And I've given hundreds of thousands of adjustments in my professional lifetime!

There have been many, many people healed through and as a result of these safe adjustments. I give all the healing credit to innate intelligence and God.

The last concern for most people is they will have to keep coming back forever. This is not true. Once you've achieved your health goal, the choice is purely up to you.

Whether or not you continue to benefit from chiropractic is basically *a choice* between sicknesscare and true healthcare. Either way, I respect your health choice, because I respect *you.*

It is my prediction that once you have increased your health, you'll go through a paradigm shift. You'll be a different person on the inside as well as the outside.

No longer will life be symptomatic or reactive based. You will choose to be a healthier, well and proactive being.

Health and wellness will have a whole new meaning to you. *And so will life!*

Welcome to the new you! May God Bless You!

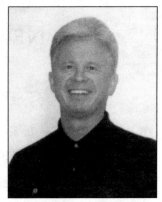

Dr. Robert R. Mariner, B.S., D.C.
Mariner Chiropractic Auto Accident
and Wellness Care Center
160 Versailles Road
Frankfort, Kentucky 40601
(502) 695-4455
DrMariner@prodigy.net
www.marinerchiropractic.com

"When health is absent,
Wisdom cannot become manifest,
Strength cannot be exerted,
Wealth is useless,
Reason is powerless."
— Herophiles 300 B.C.

"Next to God and family,
There is no greater thing in life,
Than your health!"
— Dr. Robert Mariner 2000 A.D.

Dr. Robert Mariner holds a Bachelor of Science Degree in Human Biology as well as a Doctorate of Chiropractic. He has lectured nationally and internationally on the benefits of chiropractic care. Dr. Mariner is a professionally published co-author. He is a past collegiate instructor of Anatomy and Physiology to nursing and pre-med students at Midway College, Kentucky's only all female college. Dr. Robert Mariner previously hosted the television talk show, *Your Health Matters.* He has been interviewed on radio and cable T.V. concerning the importance of chiropractic for one's overall health and well-being.

Dr. Mariner is available for private appointments or to speak locally, nationally and internationally to your club, group or organization concerning the benefits of nutrition and chiropractic. You can contact him at (502) 695-4455.

PART SIX

A New Beginning

⤜⤛

Dr. Rob Scott, M.Sc., D.C., Ph.D.(c)

*"We shall for the first time in the history of medicine
teach what I believe is the most important
subject of all — prevention of disease!"*
— Elizabeth Blackwell, M.D. 1821-1910

On October 21, 1997, my mother died after years of fighting cardiovascular disease. She was 69 years old. While she was the center of my family's world, she was but one of the millions of people who die each year from heart disease, diabetes, stroke or other chronic diseases.

Each one of the millions is a mother, a wife, a husband, sister or brother. Each one as special to their families as my mother was to mine.

The sad truth is that our country is in a health crisis. A large number of people suffer from various chronic, debilitating, lifestyle-related conditions despite our nation's increased spending on "healthcare."

According to an Associated Press report by Mark Sherman, "Healthcare spending in the United States grew to an estimated $1.7 trillion in 2003."

The United States has among the highest infant mortality rates, ranking 27th among industrialized nations. This is despite spending $5,267 per person on healthcare — well above the $2,144 per person average of other industrialized countries.

To add insult to injury, the number of deaths related to medical accident is now, according to a report by Dr. Barbara Starfield, M.D., published in the *Journal of American Medical Association*, occuring at such an alarming rate it is considered the third leading cause of death in the U.S. behind cardiovascular disease and cancer! The very system intended to make our communities healthier is now becoming a large part of the problem it was intended to solve.

Where does the problem to our health crisis lie?

Certainly it does not lie with the intentions of the men and women who work in our hospitals and health clinics. The doctors, nurses, and technicians who look after our sick are caring and compassionate individuals.

The problem lies with the model of health on which the system is built and doctors, nurses and technicians serve. The conventional model of healthcare is not a model centered on creating, improving or optimizing one's health. Rather, it is a model centered on providing care for those who are already sick.

If we truly desire to create a nation that is healthy, vivacious and free of disease, I believe we must seek a solution based on a model other than the one from which the sick care crisis arose. We must choose a healthcare model that promotes the attainment of a state of optimal health for each and every person. It must be a model that allows one to be counseled, cared for and coached to new levels of health – to levels of optimal wellness.

Thankfully, such a model of health already exists. For the past 109 years chiropractors have been educating and caring for those seeking health and wellness.

Chiropractic is a model of healthcare positioned to lead communities into the wellness revolution. The power of the chiropractic approach to health is based on physiological facts.

The chiropractic approach to health is premised on the inherent self-healing nature of the body — an ability primarily controlled and regulated through the nervous system. If for any reason there is interference with the nervous system, the body's ability to heal could be compromised.

A compromised nervous system results in what Doctors of Chiropractic refer to as dis-ease, or a lack of ease within the body. The role of the chiropractor is therefore to restore ease, once again allowing the body to optimally express health as it was designed to do.

Interference to the nervous system may come in several forms. Of importance to the chiropractor is the subluxation. A subluxation occurs when any of the movable joints of the body, primarily those of the spine, move out of their normal alignments. When this occurs it could interfere with the transmission of nerve impulses and the healing forces carried over the nerves to the organs and tissues of the body.

The easiest way to think of the effect of subluxation on nerve interference is to compare it to your cellular phone. When you are out in the open, your phone receives its full signal. It is easy to communicate clearly. However, if you are inside a building or in a place where the signal is obstructed, your communication is disrupted. Your message is not received clearly.

Subluxation could interfere with your body's signal and its ability to communicate clearly with itself. In restoring normal communication, the chiropractor's primary role is to identify and correct the nerve interference caused by subluxation.

The concept of restoring nerve system function is significant in the chiropractic model of health and wellness. It is generally accepted that three major stressors affect the onset of subluxation. These include physical, biochemical and psychological stressors.

Physical stressors could go undetected for prolonged periods of time. They could begin as early as the birthing process for a newborn. They could be as innocuous as your toddler falling in his or her efforts to walk. A physical stressor could be as traumatic as being jolted in your car by a rear end accident. One must realize that physical stressors occur daily in our lives and could unknowingly result in subluxation and nerve interference.

Biochemical stressors are all around us. In the air we breathe, the water we drink and the processed and refined foods we eat daily. It is very difficult to eliminate all the biochemical stressors entering our bodies. However, by eating whole organic foods, eliminating beverages containing artificial ingredients and avoiding areas of poor air quality one may dramatically reduce this common cause of subluxation.

Psychological stress is another common occurrence in our lives. Stress however, can be a good thing. When it is, it is called eustress. Eustress is often the driving force that allows one to perform at their peak. You have probably experienced eustress when you performed well on a test, gave a great presentation at work or played well in a big game. It is the fine balance existing between adrenaline and preparation that allows you to do well in a given situation.

My guess is, however, you have probably also experienced too much stress, or distress, where you choked and performed very poorly. In this instance, the balance shifted. Adrenaline overpowers your preparation. You can't think or perform to the best of your ability.

Distress is all too common in our lives. With fast-paced lifestyles and family and work demands, people are constantly over stressed. When one has too much stress, it becomes a negative influence and may commonly result in subluxation and nerve interference.

Traditional approaches to promoting health have included the need for exercise, nutrition and stress reduction. Each plays an important role in providing the body with needed components to function optimally. However, in the absence of proper nerve function due to subluxation, the body may not be in a position to maximize the benefit it could otherwise achieve from exercise, the nutrients it absorbs or from reduced stress.

Through an approach to restoring proper nerve function by correcting subluxations, one may ensure his or her body is able to optimally express health and the benefits from proper nutrition, exercise and stress reduction. This is the central value of chiropractic and why wellnesscare excluding chiropractic is not truly wellnesscare.

I often wonder how my mother's life would have turned out if she had been under chiropractic care since she was a child. I know from my experience as a chiropractor if she had been checked regularly for subluxation the quality of her life would have been much better, if not longer. Had there been a chiropractor to clear her nervous system from interference and to counsel, care and coach her toward reaching her desired health goals, the outcome may have been quite different.

My mother's results are no different than the majority of people who attempt to modify their health behaviors. Everybody knows smoking is bad for health; yet, many won't stop. People know exercise is good for them; yet, they won't start.

Your chiropractor can help. Allow him or her to work with you to achieve your goals. Allow your chiropractor to counsel, care and coach you to new levels of health – to a life of optimal wellness.

We know after 109 years that chiropractic has had profound positive impact on the quality of people's lives. Today, many professional athletes, movie stars and business moguls give praise to chiropractic care as a part of their successes.

This book contains many stories of the truly amazing effects chiropractic care has had on people like you and others in your community. People who have already experienced the miracle of improved health, happiness and even prosperity through chiropractic care.

I wish I could turn back time. If I could, I would ensure my mother had received the benefits of chiropractic care throughout her life. Unfortunately, that is not possible. Now that she is gone, she is a presence I feel every day in my heart and memories. Fortunately, however, it is not too late for you to start a new beginning and achieve improved levels of health through chiropractic.

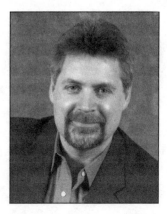

Dr. Rob Scott, M.Sc., D.C., Ph.D.(c)
Northwestern College of Chiropractic
2501 West 84th Street
Bloomington, Minnesota 55431
(952) 886-7582

Dr. Rob Scott has over 20 years experience in the health and wellness field as an exercise physiologist, chiropractor and educator. For the past five years, Dr. Scott has helped develop and instruct innovative new graduate-level courses in Integrative Health and Wellness at Northwestern Health Sciences University. He has consulted for industry in the area of worksite wellness and ergonomics in addition to a variety of other health related topics. As a practicing chiropractor, Dr. Scott is the Dean of Northwestern College of Chiropractic and is a Ph.D. candidate at the University of Minnesota. A sought after speaker, Dr. Scott has lectured internationally to a wide range of audiences on chiropractic and strategies for achieving new levels of physical and mental well-being. Dr. Scott is a member of the International Chiropractors Association and American Chiropractic Association.

To arrange for Dr. Scott to speak to your corporation, association or group, call (952) 886-7582.

CHAPTER TWO

DOCTOR APPROVED
HEALTH SECRET

PART ONE

WELLNESS: A NATURAL FEELING THROUGH CHIROPRACTIC

Dr. Patrick St. Germain, D.C.

When chiropractors are asked about chiropractic, they often begin with a personal note describing their own early experiences with chiropractic. Sometimes it is a friend or family member's life-changing experience. Other times it is a personal life-changing, miraculous moment. This may have been a turning point in the chiropractor's life, the moment destiny called out to him or her. It is with this same energy and brilliance that my own direction in life began.

When I was eight years old, I fell off my bike and suffered a concussion. Because of that fall, I suffered from debilitating headaches for the next 17 years. The headaches became more frequent and intense as I grew older.

Since my mother was a nurse, I had access to the latest and greatest medications and medical doctors. But nothing seemed to work. The headaches continued to wreak havoc on my life all the way through high school.

I was distracted by pain. Its intensity prevented me from competing at my best in school sports and activities. I was told to accept the pain. Nothing could be done to help me.

After high school graduation, I chose dentistry for my lifetime career. However, my life changed forever one summer during the in-between years of college. I injured my back working at a landscaping company. A friend recommended I see a chiropractor for my back injury. From that moment on, my entire life changed.

After only one visit, my back pain and headaches dissolved immediately. I haven't had a headache since. Not only did the chiropractor, a different kind of doctor than I was used to, relieve my pain. He also changed my life. The visit was so inspiring, I decided to change my career path and commit myself to becoming a chiropractor.

Chiropractic: Making A Difference For Those Around Me

As a chiropractor, I am making a big difference to those who suffer from headaches and backaches as well as those suffering from neck, arm, shoulder, leg and hip pains. With regular chiropractic spinal adjustments, a preventative form of healthcare, patients could live active, vibrant lives with less pain.

Over one hundred years ago, the first chiropractic adjustment was given by Dr. Daniel David Palmer to Harvey Lillard. Harvey was a janitor who had complained of hearing problems for over 17 years. Dr. Palmer found a lump in Harvey's back and suspected a vertebra was out of place. The doctor repositioned the vertebra with a gentle thrust. Much of Harvey's hearing returned after several similar treatments.

Since then, the study of this new care and the impact of impinged nerves have progressed dramatically. Years of thorough and exhaustive scientific research, testing and data resulted in the creation of universally accredited and accepted chiropractic colleges and universities. These colleges and universities are now teaching the art of chiropractic throughout the world.

With millions of patient visits since then, chiropractic has become one of the fastest growing alternative forms of healthcare in the world. I believe as more and more people concerned about their health look for a more natural and safer form of healthcare, they are turning to chiropractic.

Could Spinal Misalignment Be The Cause Of Health Problems?

In the early years, it was discovered that when the spine becomes misaligned, there could be a pinching of the nerves between the bones of the spinal column, exiting to all parts of the body. We call these pinched nerves, vertebral subluxations.

Many things could cause pinched nerves or subluxations. From trauma occurring in day-to-day home, school or work activities, injuries from amateur and professional sports, or injuries sustained in auto accidents.

One often overlooked source of subluxation is the act of being born. The birthing process places a tremendous amount of pressure on the spine and is often referred to as our first subluxation. I see a number of new parents who visit chiropractors shortly after delivering their newborns.

Subluxation Dis-ease

When the flow of nerve energy from the brain to the different parts of the body is disrupted and diminished, it could result in loss of body function. It may result in pain and dis-ease — the body no longer being at ease. This pain could be felt immediately or take years to be noticed, sometimes after it is too late to do anything about it.

When I fell off my bike at eight years old, a subluxation was created in my spine that choked off the energy flow through my nerves to parts of my body. My body was operating at less than 100 percent.

It wasn't only the pain, but also the fatigue and loss of energy preventing me from being at peak wellness.

Chiropractors: Specialists In Vertebral Subluxations

Chiropractors are the only doctors specifically trained to locate and treat spinal misalignments or subluxations. Chiropractors use their hands to apply gentle and specific pressure to the spinal column, with the goal of removing these subluxations.

Realigning the spine allows vital nerve energy the ability to reach out to every part of body.

The wonderful thing about the body is it is an amazing self-healing entity. This energy called innate intelligence is unlike anything known to man. Another important difference about chiropractic is that it doesn't just treat symptoms of pain or discomfort. Its main goal is to help correct the cause of the problem.

Chiropractic does not utilize dangerous drugs or surgery to accomplish its goals. It works with the body's own innate ability to heal itself. I feel patients who come in for regular chiropractic care know the benefits.

Some people seem to think pain is the only reason to visit a chiropractor. This thought process could be dangerous. Vertebral subluxations are often painless and could remain in you, interfering with your health for months or years before symptoms finally appear.

Pain or obvious symptoms could often be a last stage of disease. For example, would you go to a dentist who would wait until you were in pain before he checked you for cavities? An internist who told you to wait until you had a stroke before addressing high blood pressure? An oncologist who said the only time to deal with cancer was when the tumors started making you feel sick? I'm sure you get the picture.

I believe the time to correct subluxations is now! Before pain or other symptoms develop.

You may have subluxations without any spinal, nerve or muscular symptoms. My patients consider it a blessing in disguise when I am checking their spines. They say, "Wow, what did you touch? I had no idea I had a problem there. I wasn't feeling any pain."

Wellness: A Life Sustaining Commitment

My commitment to educating myself about chiropractic care and wellness has been among the most rewarding things I have ever done. This commitment has not only changed my life, but has also affected the lives of my family, my patients and my community.

I discovered there were many people in my community who didn't know about the benefits of chiropractic care. It has become my crusade to pass on this knowledge to people around me and to help them achieve overall wellness.

Wellness, in my opinion, is not just eating right, getting regular chiropractic care or managing stress. It is a combination of all of these things and more. Removing subluxations may allow the body to utilize foods more efficiently and help the body to function at 100 percent capacity.

There is a misconception among some patients. After they find relief from the pain that brought them to our office, there is no need to return to our office until they are in pain again. Fortunately, a majority of my new patients are inspired to use chiropractic care as a pathway to overall wellness.

Patient Education Making A Difference

Education is critical to understanding and achieving wellness. We spend a lot of time educating our patients about the damaging effects of vertebral subluxations. By educating patients about the benefits of spinal healthcare, they are more informed and likely to follow treatment plans.

I show patients what a healthy spine looks like. I also perform a thorough examination and take X-rays of their spines, if needed. When this is done, we begin the journey to identify the underlying cause of their respective pain and give them choices as to what could be done about their condition.

In my practice, the first approach with my patients is pain management. Pain relief is the most important thing to those in pain. After relief is attained, we start on the path to wellness. A number of our patients are tired of taking pills and potions that may not work to correct their problems, but serve only to mask the symptoms making their lives miserable.

We Treat More Than Back And Neck Conditions

Research has shown that chiropractic could benefit people of all ages and multiple conditions.

Dr. Leboeuf-Yde and others completed a study of chiropractic patients entitled *The Types and Frequencies of Improved Nonmusculoskeletal Symptoms Reported After Chiropractic Spinal Manipulative Therapy* published in *Journal of Manipulative and Physiological Therapeutic,* 1999; 22(9):559-564.

In this study, 1,504 patients were surveyed on their experiences with chiropractic care. Although many patients came in for back and neck conditions, after chiropractic care, 26 percent of patients reported improvements related to airway passages (usually reported as "easier to breathe"); 25 percent of patients reported improvements related to the digestive system (mostly reported as "improved function"); 14 percent of patients reported improvements in eyes/vision (usually reported as "improved vision"); and 14 percent reported improvements in heart/circulation (about half of these reported as "improved circulation").

According to an article on this study by the Maine Chiropractic Association, "Of patients treated in one spinal area 15 percent had a non-musculosketal benefit. In two spinal areas the percentage increased to 22 percent. With (spinal treatment in) three areas 32 percent (reported improvements) and with four (treatments areas of the spine) 35 percent (reported health improvements beyond bone, joint and muscles)."

Sound too good to be true? Consider the fact that nerve energy flows from the brain through the spinal column to all parts of the body. Every function of the body follows this flow of energy and could be affected by spinal subluxations.

New data has reported even minor pressure on nerves exiting the spine could cause problems. These could go undetected for years and lead to long-term health problems.

A review of literature entitled *The Effects of Mild Compression on Spinal Nerve Roots With Implications for Models of Verte-*

bral Subluxation and the Clinical Effects of Chiropractic Adjustment: A Review of the Literature by Dr. Scott Alderson and Dr. George Muhs published in the *Journal of Vertebral Subluxation Research* adds further evidence to what many Doctors of Chiropractic have known for years.

Commenting on this research, Dr. Matthew McCoy, editor of the *Journal of Vertebral Subluxation Research* said, "This review of literature is extremely comprehensive in nature and adds a mountain of evidence...Subluxations don't always cause symptoms and that the longer you have them the worse they get and the more difficult they are to correct. This is another strong argument for having children checked by chiropractors at a young age for vertebral subluxation."

Chiropractic has made a difference in my life and is making a positive difference in the lives of all of my patients. This simple theory about nerve interference has come a long way in improving the lives of people in my office and millions of people around the world. The journey to good health is not a quick or easy one. It is all about knowledge. Knowledge is power. By educating patients of their options, we offer them a chance at a new beginning, new hope and, most of all, help in attaining a desirable and beneficial state of wellness.

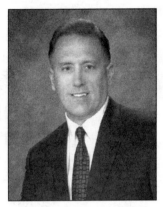

Dr. Patrick St. Germain, D.C.
St. Germain Chiropractic, P.A.
877 S. Orange Blossom Trail,
Apopka, Florida
(407) 889-3223
www.stgermainchiropractic.com

He didn't know it at the time, but his bicycle injury as a young boy would lead him to his future role and love as a chiropractic health giver. After his bicycle injury, he suffered with headache misery for 17 years before a miraculous experience with a chiropractor changed his life forever.

Dr. St. Germain would also discover miracles are a daily experience for him and others in the chiropractic profession because of the incredible power of the human body to heal. A power unlocked with the assistance of Doctors of Chiropractic, who find and correct spinal subluxations and pinched nerves that could impede and restrict the flow of vital nerve energy from the brain to all parts of the body.

Dr. Patrick has been spreading the chiropractic message throughout central Florida for over 15 years. He has helped thousands of people to regain their health and, through his wellness clinics, has helped them to also maintain their good health.

Dr. Patrick St. Germain, D.C. is the Founder and Director of St. Germain Chiropractic, P.A. with offices in Apopka, Kissimmee and Winter Garden, Florida. He specializes in wellnesscare including adult and pediatric care, job related injuries and auto accident injuries. He is a graduate of Life Chiropractic College in Marietta, Georgia and holds a Master's Degree in Biomechanical Trauma. Dr. St. Germain is also a Certified Independent Forensic Chiropractic Medical Examiner.

His main office is located at 877 S. Orange Blossom Trail, Apopka, Florida. If you would like to schedule a private appointment with Dr. St. Germain, find out more about his clinics or arrange for Dr. St. Germain to speak to your corporation or group, he can be reached at (407) 889-3223 or visit his web site at www.stgermainchiropractic.com.

PART TWO

CHIROPRACTIC AND THE IMMUNE SYSTEM

❦

Dr. Jack Thompson, B.S., D.C.

When I started my formal training at Life Chiropractic University, I took hundreds of hours of anatomy, physiology and other medical courses to prepare me to practice as a Primary Care Physician. After speaking with many practicing chiropractors, especially older ones with many years of experience, I became fascinated by the types of problems that improved as a result of the spinal treatments rendered by the chiropractor.

I heard stories of patients being relieved from headaches and back pain. Other stories seemed impossible to me. But I was intrigued, so I listened. They told me about a patient with chronic heartburn whose symptoms were alleviated after spinal care. One older chiropractor told me a story about World War 1. Before antibiotics many soldiers died of infections related to battle wounds. These poor souls were housed in a holding area until they passed away because it was felt nothing more could be done for them.

The story goes that there was a chiropractor who would secretly, at night, give spinal adjustments to these soldiers. To the amazement of the medical staff some of these men began to recover from infection.

Now, I thought this was an interesting and entertaining story.

It had me wondering, "If this has a thread of truth, how in the world could chiropractic care help with infections?"

Incredible System

Here is what I have come to believe. Our bodies have a built in "defense system" called the immune system. The immune system continuously monitors our entire body. It sends out specific cells to fight off and kill "invader cells" or other bad cells. If we cut a finger, for example, the immune system sends specific white blood cells. These engulf and destroy dirt particles, germs, bacteria or virus organisms that may have entered the body via the cut. Pus, which builds up around a cut, is actually the product of the white blood cells destroying these invader microorganisms.

Our bodies have many levels of defense and "weapons" to protect us. Skin and mucous membranes create physical barriers to invasion. Digestive juices dissolve germs. Urine cleans the urinary tract. Skin secretions kill many germs before they can ever enter into the body. Fevers burn off microorganisms. Swelling helps clean out an area. Specialized white blood cells attack and devour intruders. Macrophages, T cells, killer cells, lymphocytes, antibodies and other specialized cells each have their own specific functions aimed at killing and removing potentially harmful cells from our bodies.

There are also specialized organ systems producing these defensive cells — bone marrow, spleen, thymus, tonsils, adenoids, appendix and lymph nodes — all of which are extremely important to our overall health.

What's not commonly understood is that what has a power for good can have a potential for bad.

An unhealthy immune system can overreact as an allergic or hypersensitivity reaction. It can under-react as immune deficiency disorders. It can attack the very body it was meant to serve.

Controlling Immune System

Our brain and nerves provide communication control of the immune system. The brain and the nerves send signals from the body to the brain and back again, controlling and coordinating our body functions.

I believe the quality and quantity of these signals running over the nerves to and from the brain need to be optimal to allow the brain to have the highest level of communication with the systems in the body.

For over 109 years, chiropractors have made it their area of expertise to diagnosis and treat a condition known as vertebral subluxation. This is where spinal bones "lock-up," causing pressure on the delicate spinal nerves or even on the lower portion of the brain itself.

By restoring motion to spinal bones, the chiropractor removes dangerous nerve pressure. This could allow the brain to receive more accurate information from the nerves monitoring all parts of the body.

With more accurate information, doesn't it make sense that the responses given out by the brain and carried by the nerve system are more timely and appropriate for establishing a state of optimal health in the body?

As nerve pressure is released, could an overall strengthening and healing of many systems of the body begin to occur?

I believe a strong immune system is the utmost requirement for optimal health. The immune system is at work everywhere throughout the body. As it grows stronger, the body's ability to fight infectious illness begins to increase.

Better Health

Speaking for myself, my immune system changed radically for the better when I started receiving regular chiropractic spinal care.

When I was in my thirties, I had a terrible history of chronic migraine headaches, sometimes three to four per week. I also would get common colds about four times per year and they would take about ten days to completely resolve. The colds always started with sore throats, which turned into sinus congestion and finally resulted in severe bronchitis. I could count the progression of the cold like clockwork. At about ten days or so, they would finally resolve.

After about four weeks and approximately twelve chiropractic spinal care appointments, I noticed my headaches had decreased dramatically. As the months of chiropractic care continued, I noticed I did not get the usual head colds I had been plagued with for years!

To my amazement, to this day, I no longer get the dreadful migraine headaches. To my greatest pleasure, I no longer catch my ten-day common cold.

As far as I'm concerned, the ability to ward off my common cold could only have happened through the strengthening of my immune system.

Now, after more than fourteen years of continuous chiropractic spinal care, I can tell you I rarely catch the flu or any other type of common infection. I have not taken an antibiotic for an infectious ailment in that entire time. And I have never felt better or healthier than I do today.

Doesn't it just make sense that if the brain and nerve system have less pressure and are working better, all the systems of the body could be able to work better?

Health And Harmony

Doctors of Chiropractic analyze the spine to locate misaligned spinal bones, a condition known as vertebral subluxation. This condition could cause spinal distortions and interference with the function of the brain and nerve systems.

The exact mechanism of how the nervous system interacts with the immune system is one of the hottest areas of scientific inquiry. This new field is called "psychoneuroimmunology."

I hope I have opened your eyes to some new and truly revolutionary concepts in health and healing. I believe, and it has been my personal experience, that keeping the spine moving freely by receiving routine Chiropractic spinal care is one of the best ways to keep your brain and nerve system free of interference. I feel this allows more optimal control of all of the systems of the body.

Doesn't it make sense that when all your body's systems are working optimally, and in harmony with each other, you could enjoy overall optimal health?

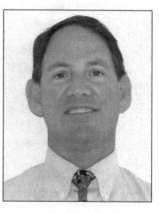

Dr. Jack R. Thompson, B.S., D.C.
Synergy Chiropractic Wellness Center
305 Hanson Avenue, Suite. 160
Fredericksburg, Virginia 22401
phone (540) 310-4930
fax (540) 310-4938
email jrtchiro@hotmail.com

After graduating high school in St. Augustine, Florida, Dr. Jack Thompson attended the University of Central Florida where he earned a Bachelor of Science degree in Electrical Engineering in 1978. He worked as a Senior Scientist for AT&T for eight years. Then as Project Manager for the Institute for Simulation and Training in Orlando, Florida for four years before discovering the wonders of chiropractic in 1989. In 1990, he decided to obtain his Doctorate of Chiropractic degree. In 1995, he graduated number one in his class (Valedictorian) and has owned and operated a successful practice since.

Dr. Thompson believes people are "hungry" for the common sense message of chiropractic. His practice focuses on family wellness and preventative care. He believes education is the best way to teach the importance of proper spinal function in the restoration and maintenance of health. Dr. Thompson has written numerous health related articles for local publications. He enjoys his family, boating and flying. He says that his wife and life partner, Debra, is the sole reason for his success.

To schedule a private appointment with Dr. Thompson or to arrange for Dr. Thompson to speak to your corporation or group, call (540) 310-4930.

PART THREE

HAVE WE OVERLOOKED THE KEY TO HEALTH?

❦

Dr. Douglas Wine, D.C

Thank you for picking up this book. In doing so, you have taken a different approach and a good attitude towards your health. You have also just taken a huge step toward obtaining the ultimate goal, which is optimal health.

In this book, you will read about the fabulous benefits, the different techniques and all other aspects of the chiropractic profession. These chapters relate to how chiropractic helps all different types of people, some of them children, some elderly — all of them just "normal" everyday people.

You will read about everything from headaches, asthma, sports injuries to all other aspects of health. But most importantly, what you are going to read in this chapter will lay the foundation for everything else you read in this book.

Have we overlooked the simplicity of our health? Don't get me wrong. I am not saying the human body is anything simple. The human body is very complex. In fact, it is the most complex thing on earth.

Imagine inviting the most acclaimed scientists in the world to a laboratory asking them to bring their computers, machines and any other equipment they would like. Then, we hand the scientists hamburgers, french fries and sodas asking them to covert these foods into any human body tissue they could. The scientists would not be able to make one living cell. Yet the human body does this by design on its own all by itself consistently during an entire lifetime.

However, we take all of that for granted.

Systems Of The Body

How does the human body function? There are twelve major systems in the human body. These systems are the skeletal, muscular, circulatory, respiratory, digestive, lymphatic, immune, sensory, urinary, reproductive, endocrine and central nerve systems. Of these twelve systems, the central nerve system controls all other eleven. If there were any interference in that primary system, then automatically one or more of the other eleven systems could be affected.

For example, take one room in your home in which you have different systems such as lights, computer, television, heater, fan, radio, etc. Let's say all these different systems are working in that particular room. If all those systems suddenly shut down, what would be the first thing that you would do? You would check the electrical breaker system because it controls the flow to all of those other systems in that particular room. You certainly would not start by changing all of the light bulbs or by buying a new computer, new radio or a new fan before checking that primary system, the breaker system.

So wouldn't it make sense if something in the human body started to malfunction, logically, the first thing to be checked would be the number one system? Wouldn't it make even more sense to properly maintain your primary nervous system to insure the other 11 systems function properly at all times to avoid unnecessary problems in the future?

The central nerve system consists of the brain and spinal cord. It controls 100 percent of everything else going in the human body. Here are some other amazing things about that central nerve system.

First To Form

When a man and a woman come together to conceive a baby, the first group of cells that actually develop in the womb are the brain cells. After there are a certain number of these brain cells, there is a small extension that starts to develop which is termed the spinal cord. Once that has developed to a certain proportion, there are branches that start to appear at multiple levels. This is the start of the peripheral nerve system. At the end of those branches all the other different tissues of the human body start to develop.

First the brain and spinal cord have to produce the life force, intelligence and blue prints before any other tissues of the human body can start to be manufactured.

The second amazing thing about the brain and spinal cord (central nerve system) is they are the only parts of the human body that seem to have to last us our entire lifetime. Once we are at the age of approximately two to three years old, we have all the central nerve system cells we will ever have for the rest of our lives. The other tissues of the body, including the peripheral nerve system, continue to regenerate automatically our entire lifetime.

Another amazing fact is the central nerve system is the only organ in the human body that is entirely protected by bone. The brain is completely surrounded by the skull and the spinal cord is fully encased by the vertebrae. At every level of those vertebrae is where the peripheral nerves exit and communicate with all of the other 70 thousand trillion cells of the human body allowing them to develop, function and regenerate. Interference in that communication could create dis-ease.

The Key To Health

If any of these twelve systems lose their ability to contribute their share of function, all of the cells of the body suffer. Extreme dysfunction could lead to death whereas moderate dysfunction could lead to sickness.

Do you know what factor is used to determine life from death? In order to be pronounced dead, the brain has no more electrical impulses. Therefore, if the brain is communicating at 100 percent with all the other tissues of the human body, you are 100 percent alive. If the brain does not communicate at all with the other cells, you are 100 percent dead. If there is any interference with the communication from the brain to any other living body tissues, then could it be said the body is proportionally dead or alive, relative to the amount of interference?

For example, if I go into your shoulder and completely sever the nerve, your entire arm would go dead. You would not feel it, move it, nor would there be any function or regeneration.

But if only 25 percent of the nerve were choked off, would that mean your arm was 75 percent alive, but 25 percent dead? The same scenario exists for every organ, every gland, every muscle and every other tissue of the human body. If the nerve system is able to communicate at 100 percent with all of those body tissues, then you are 100 percent alive. If there is any interference, whatever percent of interference exists is how much life force you lose to that particular area which, in turn, could compromise your full health potential.

The principal area in the human body where communication interference between the central nerve system and the rest of the body occurs is at the vertebral level. When any vertebra moves out of its normal position, it could place pressure on the nerve, which in turn could interfere with communication.

That vertebral interference is called a subluxation. Subluxations are, therefore, directly proportional to your health. The body is a fabulous machine. It needs no help. It just needs no interference.

I believe the best chance you have in your entire lifetime to be healthy is to make sure that there is no interference in your nerve system. If subluxation exists, you could be automatically compromising your health. Chiropractic is the only profession dedicating itself entirely to finding and correcting subluxations.

Luck Or Chiropractic?

When I am asked how my family is doing, my response is always the same: "My family is very healthy, thank you."

You see, my oldest daughter is 18 years old. She has never been sick a day in her life. She has never had a cold or flu, an allergy or a headache. In fact, she has never had so much as an aspirin in her body. So I must be very lucky. I also have a 16-year-old son. He's never been sick a day in his life. Never a cold or flu, an allergy or a headache. He has never had so much as an aspirin in his body. I must be incredibly lucky. And I have a 13-year-old daughter with the same scenario. She has never needed any kind of chemical or drug. I must be the luckiest man alive.

But wait. My wife, whom I have been with for over 30 years has never had any health issues or any typical female problems such as menstrual cramps. She has had no reason to put any toxins in her body. I also have a dog. He's four years old and never had a reason to go to the vet. I happen to be 49-years-old, have never been sick a day in my life and have never missed a day of work.

My entire family, including Aldo, our dog, has been under chiropractic care our entire lives. I was fortunate to have parents who were under chiropractic care and, in turn, I have been under chiropractic care since birth. My wife has been under chiropractic care since we began dating. Each of my children has been adjusted regularly since day one. The fact is I have an extraordinarily healthy family.

Is it coincidence or is it chiropractic?

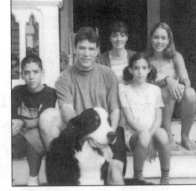

Dr. Douglas Wine, D.C.
Wine Chiropractic
58 Winnacunnet Road
Hampton, New Hampshire 03842
(603) 929-5000
www.winechiropractic.com

Dr. Douglas Wine has been enhancing health through chiropractic for over two decades in Europe and the United States. While in Europe for 14 years he earned the reputation of being one of the foremost chiropractors in France and Switzerland. Dr. Wine's successful practice has included top ranked European athletes on the Swiss Olympic team in addition to French national soccer players and the Tour de France cyclists. Celebrities, government officials and politicians, police and fire department employees and their families have all selected Dr. Wine for their personal chiropractic care. In his 24 years of practice, Dr. Wine has personally cared for over 35,000 different patients.

Dr. Wine is highly regarded by his colleagues as a mentor in his field having professionally taught the chiropractic technique and philosophy throughout the United States and Europe. Complementing his highly effective chiropractic style, he is recognized and respected for is his candid ability to effectively explain health issues in a variety of ways to all age groups from toddlers to seniors. He has a unique ability to connect with people from all walks of life with wit and laughter while maintaining professional integrity. Watch for Dr. Wine's upcoming books.

To obtain a wealth of health information please visit www.winechiropractic.com . To schedule a private appointment with Dr. Wine or arrange for Dr. Wine to speak to your corporation or group, call (603) 929-5000.

PART FOUR

Two Worlds Collide

Dr. Matthew Bateman B.Sc, G. Dip.Ed, M.Chiro.
Dr. Bridie Cullinane B.App.Sc, B.Chiro.Sc

It took less than a second to change my life. It could have been a second that never happened…

At 16 years of age, she finished drinking the one litre of water she had been instructed to drink before her ultrasound scheduled in just a few hours. She walked over and collapsed on the couch. This had become an all too familiar occurrence. The young woman wondered how many more times she would need to endure this procedure before she and her parents would agree with their doctor's advice to surgically remove one or both ovaries.

A few days later, the young woman had the results. It was the same outcome as all the other times. A large cyst growing on her ovary. This time on the left side. She did not know it yet, but this would prove to be the last time she would have to endure embarrassing, painful tests and get the same demoralizing results. Soon this vicious cycle would end.

One month later, late at night, she hungrily went to the refrigerator. After reaching deep inside the refrigerator shelves, the young woman stood up and hit her shoulder. The impact shocked her. She paused for a few minutes to catch her breath.

The blow to the shoulder hurt, but it seemed relatively insignificant at the time. Far from being insignificant, it was an event that would change her life forever.

The next day, she developed a dull ache in her middle back.

It gradually worsened until the pain was so severe even breathing brought tears to her eyes.

A friend noticed. After an explanation, the friend immediately produced the phone number of her chiropractor saying, "Call him. He'll be able to help you."

The 16-year-old girl wasn't completely convinced. She had reservations about visiting a chiropractor. But desperate times called for desperate measures. She decided to give him a call.

After a thorough examination, the chiropractor explained the young woman had subluxations in her middle back. She was informed by her chiropractor the subluxations were blocking the healing forces meant to be flowing through her nervous system. She was also told of a subluxation in her lower back. This was an area where she had not experienced pain. She was told it was the exact area suppling nerve flow to the reproductive organs. She was in shock. The young woman had not even told the chiropractor about her ovarian cysts. She believed the cysts were not something a chiropractor could help her with.

The pain in the middle back went away after just two adjustments. With chiropractic care, the ovarian cysts dissolved progressively. One year after her first adjustment, there was no sign of the ovarian cysts and no need for the surgery that may have left her incapable of having children.

My name is Dr. Bridie Cullinane. I know this story well because I was the 16-year-old girl you just read about. Chiropractic care changed my life forever. Two years after my first visit to the chiropractor, I moved over 2000 km from my hometown to become a chiropractor myself.

Chiropractic care has changed my life in more ways than I could possibly express. As a child, I had an incredible temper. I drove my family crazy with my behaviour and irrationalism. I have no doubt had I been born in the 1990s, I would have been diagnosed with Attention Deficit Disorder or some other type of behavioural disorder.

From my first adjustment, my personality started to change. I no longer felt angry towards the world and was more balanced in my moods.

Every day I am grateful for chiropractic and the friend who cared enough to recommend it to me. I meet women often who were in my same situation. They took the surgical option. While deeply saddened for them, I feel hopeful chiropractic care may soon become the first option — not the last — for women who find themselves in my situation.

A World Apart

My name is Dr. Matthew Bateman.

Like Dr. Bridie, I was introduced to chiropractic by a caring friend. However, my story in chiropractic is at the other end of the health spectrum. I feel blessed I have not suffered a serious pain or illness like countless others have.

You see, my story is of a recovery that never needed to occur, of an illness that has not happened and of a life free from major health complications. I believe I am part of a growing breed at the forefront of a wellness revolution.

In my opinion, society has placed more importance on the restoration of health over the maintenance of health. We see it all the time on television shows such as *ER*. The young, dedicated doctors armed with stethoscopes and defibrillators saving lives.

In the case of accidents, a medical doctor's work is truly life saving. However, I believe far more damage occurs from the effects of chronic diseases. Heart disease is the number one killer in the world right now. Cancer is number two. Both of these killers might be preventable by living a wellness lifestyle, which includes regular chiropractic care. A wellness lifestyle is a far cry from the excitement of *ER*. It requires a different focus and commitment.

I see the real health miracle saving lives is through prevention rather than cure. I call these stories silent miracles. Silent because these are the things we don't hear about. It could be the happy, healthy child who sleeps through the night. The worker whose sick days are never taken. The athlete who remains injury free.

Peak Performance

As a patient, chiropractic care has always been about higher performance and peak potential for me. As a chiropractor, I am fortunate to work with people who excel in all walks of life. This includes elite level athletes.

Elite level athletes push the limits of what seems humanly possible. Then they discover they can push some more. As a chiropractor working with these athletes, my job is to simply help their bodies function better naturally.

However, what I am about to tell you may shock you. In sports, it is not usually the fastest athlete who wins. The winner is usually the athlete who slows down the least.

For example, look at the 100m sprint. Most athletes have the same top speed. Most reach this top speed by the 60m mark. The athlete slowing the least during the final 40m is the ultimate winner.

Compare that to life. We are now living longer than ever. In fact, in Australia the number of people living over the age of 80 is expected to triple. The number of centurions (people living to 100 years or older) is set to explode by 1500 percent over the next 50 years. For some people, the thought of living to 100 years old with the health they have — or expect to have — is simply frightening.

The Finish Line Of Life

As people contemplate their lives, most express to me that they don't want to endure years of crippling pain or illness, the loss of their friends or loved ones or the devastating effects on their minds due to dementias like Alzheimer's.

Unfortunately, some people are crawling through the last 40 meters of their lives. Due to the choices made throughout their lives, some people will end up living too short and dying too long. I believe this does not have to be the case. However, living a long, healthy life requires a decision to do just that. The earlier in life the decision is made, the better. Squeezing the very most out of life is something we all should aim to achieve.

For me, choosing a chiropractic lifestyle was easy. It just made so much sense. Why? My view is that when we were born, we innately knew how to be healthy. We didn't need to go to university to learn how to heal a cut, digest our food or direct the millions of functions our bodies attend to every second.

Two Worlds Meet

It is fitting these two chiropractors from worlds apart became united by a common vision at the start of the new millennium — better health for every body.

Imagine the possibility of a baby born into this world without needing a single medication! Imagine a child who has complete trust in his or her body's ability to remain healthy. What would you give to have a teenager easily adapt to our ever changing world? What would it mean to be an adult who is a loving, healthy and productive member of society? Now imagine what the world could be like if everyone adopted a chiropractic lifestyle.

Today, we have two fantastic practices helping people of all ages achieve optimal health. As experts in healthy living, we see incredible wellness happen in our practices every day. We believe there are many more healings we don't see.

Chiropractic is more than an adjustment to correct vertebral subluxation. Chiropractic art, science and philosophy are a way of life. While not a universal remedy for every health concern, it is a vital part of being healthy.

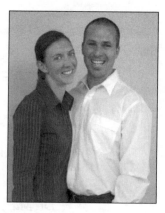

**Dr. Bridie Cullinane B.App.Sc,
B.Chiro.Sc
Dr. Matthew Bateman B.Sc,
G. Dip.Ed, M. Chiro.**
Peak Potential Health and Wellness Centres
256 Balcombe Rd
Mentone, Australia
61 3+ 9584 1308
www.peakpotential.com.au

Australia's Leaders in Health and Wellness with offices in Mentone and Bulleen, Australia.

To schedule a private appointment with either doctor or to arrange for either to speak to your corporation or group, call 61 3+ 9584 1308 or 61 3+ 9852 4555.

PART FIVE

CHIROPRACTIC MAKES PERFECT SENSE

Dr. MaryAnne Shiozawa, D.C.

How many times in your life did something make perfect sense to you? I've had many experiences as an adult where concepts and ideas felt good to me. I adopted them into my life.

But, as adults I think we are more guarded about new beliefs. As we get older, we criticize and assess more before we make decisions. We tend to gather as much information before we get to the point of accepting something into our lives.

There's something pure and innocent in children we might lose as adults. Children embrace concepts readily with open minds uninfluenced by life experiences. This is how I embraced chiropractic.

You may be reading this book because you found it on someone's coffee table. Maybe you found it in a bookstore. Perhaps someone gave it to you. You saw the title, *The World's Best Kept Health Secret Revealed*. It jarred your curiosity. What could this secret be?

I hope the answers you find in this book will transform your life to another level and provide information to expand your views on your health.

That's what this book is about…your health. The most important aspect of your life. To achieve your optimal state of health, you must embrace wellness. It is my belief chiropractic care is the path to wellness.

Discovering Chiropractic

When I was 11 years old, my little sister played on a soccer team. The parents of the players arranged for a teammate's father, Dr. Bill, to be the soccer team's chiropractor. At the field before each match, Dr. Bill would provide chiropractic care to make sure the girls' spines, joints and muscular structures were in proper alignment so the games would result in fewer or no injuries.

Even though at 11 years old I didn't fully understand the power of the care he was providing, intuitively I knew Dr. Bill was helping the girls. As a young girl, I also received regular chiropractic care to keep my body healthy.

A few years later, I babysat for Dr. Bill's family. I was fascinated by how enthusiastic and knowledgeable his kids were about living healthy and happy lives. I was inspired. As a 14-year-old, I didn't have much knowledge of healthcare. But what I learned from his family made complete sense to me. Health and wellness through chiropractic care is a lifestyle.

I made the choice to become a chiropractor when I was 14 years old.

Chiropractic Dream

I tell this story to almost all of my patients and they always respond by saying, "Wow. You knew when you were that young?" Their eyes open wide, acknowledging it is impressive and commendable. But really, I don't necessarily look at it this way. I know I didn't back when I was 14. Sure, something in me felt a powerful pull each time I thought about being a chiropractor. But as a teenager, the only thing I knew was to follow my heart. That's what kids do. They dream. And they innately follow their hearts.

As adults, the world of dreams seems harder to achieve. We doubt ourselves too much. Our egos get in the way. We're too busy proving that we're right and they're wrong. Most of us don't listen to each other anymore.

When seeing new ideas and concepts, adults might grasp them more cautiously. We believe we know enough to make our lives work. We have daily routines with our families, our careers, our diets, how we think and the activities in which we participate.

Simply put, the game of life happens. And then what? We all want the best things in life.

Where Is Your Focus?

I believe most adults have lost focus. We've confused our priorities. There are many directions in life. The most important is the one that will create a life you love filled with happiness and health.

Living a healthy, happy life is an ongoing pursuit. Perhaps, we try new ideas. We might experiment with something we discovered from a book or a conversation with a friend.

What Would Make A Difference In Your Life?

We're all on this planet for one thing...to live. How would you live your life at its best? What would you do to be your happiest? Are you living a life you love? Are you truly healthy? Could you be healthier?

As human beings, I believe we are born to be healthy. I feel an innate force exists within all living creatures driving us to live great lives of happiness, abundance and love. It could be called many names. Universal intelligence. God. Regardless of the name, I feel wellness comes from this power within. This may be a new concept for some.

A New Way Of Thinking

For you to find what you're looking for in this book, try opening your mind like a child would open his or her mind. What does that mean?

If you watch children playing and laughing you will see purity and innocence. The power of a child's mind to gather knowledge, without bias, is unmatched by most adults. Studies have shown we lose creative power as time passes.

As adults we deal with increasing amounts of information daily, which distracts from the inner voice of our universal intelligence. To overcome this feeling of separation, the moment something inspires you and speaks to your heart is the moment to embrace it. Children do this daily. Why must adults be so guarded and shielded?

Embrace who you are as a divine human being. Invite and welcome your childlike self. It's a beautiful way to live.

For me, the choice at a young age to pursue a career as a chiropractor was easy and made perfect sense. My decisions were not clouded with the increased skepticism or judgment that comes with age. As a child, chiropractic and the love of life were pure thoughts. I took the reins and held on, helping people understand their bodies and health. Learn about the benefits of chiropractic care and the devastating results if the spine isn't properly cared for.

Living Fully

Open your adult mind. Invite dreams to be fulfilled. Live the life you've always envisioned. Laugh like you did when you were a child. You just may surprise yourself. Good things will happen. Breathe a little deeper. Swing your arms when you walk. Get your blood pumping.

Go see your chiropractor. Keep your spine healthy. Bring your whole family. You and your children will smile.

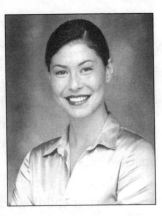

Dr. MaryAnne Shiozawa, D.C.
Shiozawa Wellness Center
3 East 44th Street, 5th Floor
New York, New York 10017
(877) 867-7477
www.wellshio.com

Dr. Shiozawa is a board certified chiropractor and owner of Shiozawa Wellness Center in New York City. With an emphasis on total body wellness through maintaining a healthy spine, Dr. Shiozawa's clients include a broad spectrum of New Yorkers, from CEOs and business owners to film stars and Broadway performers.

Dr. Shiozawa was given an honorary recognition from the New York Chiropractic Council for giving voluntary chiropractic services to the NYPD and FDNY at Ground Zero. Dr. Shiozawa is also a passionate triathlete who just finished her first Ironman distance triathlon in July 2004 in Lake Placid, New York. She plans on racing in Korea for the 2005 Ironman triathlon.

PART SIX

AMERICAN OVERDOSE

✑

Dr. Jason Gerard, D.C.

Growing up in Minnesota I dreamed of playing college hockey with the intention of pursuing a career as a professional hockey player.

After being the starting goaltender for three years and winning various awards, such as All-Conference in my senior year, I began receiving letters and visits from top college hockey programs. However, an injury I sustained during a practice for my high school football team changed the direction of my life forever.

During football practice, three months before hockey season, I jumped to catch a pass and was undercut by the defender. I landed hard on my back, was injured and had trouble breathing.

I started physical therapy with the sports trainer. Within a few weeks after the incident I started to feel better — but not great. During my therapy I was put on an asthma inhaler because I was experiencing breathing trouble. My doctor called it exercise-induced asthma. I didn't think twice about it.

The problem with the asthma inhaler was that it sped up my heart – it was like eating five candy bars. After the initial rush, my body came down hard leaving me fatigued.

A few months passed. I became more and more dependent on the inhaler. When hockey season started I was using the inhaler only at the end of games. As the season progressed, I wanted to use it every period.

The air in a hockey arena is not the best, and having asthma made it even worse. The quality of my play declined — that something extra seemed to be missing. I was fatigued and I was just 17. Interest from the top college hockey programs went away.

Chiropractic Choice

Once at college, I decided to pursue a career in sports medicine. I remembered being worked on by the trainers and thought sports medicine was a career option for me. I began contacting local chiropractors. I thought they might fit into the path of study I was pursuing.

One day, I sat watching a chiropractor adjust people. I noticed the change it made in them immediately. At the end of the day, the chiropractor came over to me and said, "I hear you wheezing. If I help you by adjusting you and getting rid of your asthma and your need for that inhaler, would you become a chiropractor?"

I said, yes, because I didn't believe he could help me. But after just one adjustment, my wheezing went away completely. He continued to adjust me. I have not used an inhaler in about 15 years.

I held up my end of the bargain. I became a chiropractor because I wanted to change peoples' lives for the better, too.

Professional Goal

As a chiropractor, I am frustrated by some current beliefs that we should look outside our bodies to medications every time we feel ill. When I opened my practice, I made it my goal to help people have another option.

This promise was put to the test by a female patient with a five-year-old son. For many months, this patient came to my office for adjustments. Her son was with her. I never asked her if he should be checked and needed care, even though I felt he did. That changed the day she came in for an adjustment without him.

I asked her why she didn't have her son with her. She pointed to the bags under her eyes and said she had just spent the past 24 hours in an emergency room with her son. He almost died from taking a medication for his ADHD that was prescribed by his doctor.

That night I went home with tears in my eyes and made a pact with myself. It would become my goal to give families — particularly families with kids – alternative healthcare and wellnesscare options.

The next time I saw this patient I told her I would check her son. It was my goal for her to have a healthy son who did not need to rely on a lifetime of drugs and medications.

As I started to adjust him, he became a changed person. His energy and vitality came back. And guess what? The doctor slowly removed him from the medication! How cool.

Options To Alternatives

It seems to me there are medications for everything. A medication if you sleep too much. A medication if you sleep too little. I believe there's a point where our culture looks at this and says, "Okay, enough is enough."

The American healthcare system is rated number 37 by the World Health Organization — a telling statistic. That puts us between Costa Rica and Slovakia in terms of quality of healthcare. Would you feel comfortable getting injured and going to a hospital in Costa Rica?

Studies show nearly 100,000 people a year die from *properly* prescribed medications.

A 50-year-old female patient of mine walked through my door with the look of somebody who was worn, like the world had fallen on top of her. During our initial interview she was not very responsive, friendly or happy. After awhile, I remarked she hadn't said much. I asked if there was something I could do to make her more comfortable.

She broke down in tears and admitted she had been to so many doctors who promised they could help. She was tired of getting the runaround and wanted to know if I could really help her. I told her I didn't know, but I was sure going to try.

The patient said she was feeling good until the age of 40 when she started to experience menopause-like symptoms. For the next five to 10 years, her doctors put her on a variety of medications. When one didn't work, they tried another. Soon, she was taking medications simply to counter the effects of other medications.

I began adjusting her. Within weeks she came out of her shell. On her own accord and not under my direction, she chose to limit her medications one at a time. She met with her medical doctor three months after starting adjustments. Her doctor told her she looked great and the medications she was taking must be working. She laughed and told him she had made the choice to stop her medications. She walked out of his office for the last time.

Since then she has brought in her whole family including her children and her grandkids. She is now an advocate that health comes from within. In my practice, I find this is a typical story. Patients find increased health and wellness and then bring in their entire families.

I believe a number of medications are for crisis care of a condition and not for wellness. Let's say you have high blood pressure. You could take a pill for the rest of your life to regulate your blood pressure. What if you asked yourself, "What might I do so I don't have to rely on this pill for the rest of my life?"

How about children? Should we just put kids on behavioral medications and not really ask why there are behavioral issues?

The goal of chiropractic is to educate people about how to achieve true wellness.

Getting Started

I give every patient a thorough and detailed examination. Afterwards I present them with a report outlining my findings. Then we sit down one-on-one and go over the report so I can answer any questions and explain the results of my exam.

I educate patients that health is about the body functioning at 100 percent — which could be more than simply being pain-free.

The moment of truth for most patients is after we've gone through the report and they look at their X-rays. The patient actually sees the spinal misalignments, degeneration and curvatures.

We are a society wanting instant results. We want things fixed now. Problems dealt with now. The pharmaceutical industry has picked up on this. I watch advertisements promoting medications offering quick fixes not requiring a lot of time or effort.

Americans are being inundated with the message about medications. I believe we need to educate people that true health and wellness could come from within our own bodies — not outside. Opponents to this belief would argue people live longer because of medications. But my response is we may live longer, but it does not mean we are living *healthier*.

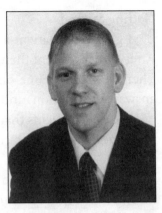

Dr. Jason Gerard, D.C.
Lakewoods Chiropractic, P.A.
255 Highway 97, Suite 2A
Forest Lake, Minnesota 55025
(651) 464-0800
www.LakeWoodsChiropractic.com

Jason Gerard, D.C. runs a busy chiropractic practice with his wife Josee Gerard, D.C. in Forest Lake, Minnesota. Lakewoods Chiropractic, P.A. was founded on the principles of quality care, even better education and, most of all, healthy chiropractic, drug-free families. Dr. Gerard can be reached at (651) 464-0800 or www.lakewoodschiropractic.com .

CHAPTER THREE

PREGNANCY AND CHILDREN HEALTH SECRET

PART ONE

WELLNESS STARTS WITH THE GLEAM IN YOUR PARENTS' EYES

❧

Dr. Claire H. O'Neill-Close, D.C., F.I.C.P.A

"The doctor of the future will give no medicine, but will interest his patients in the care of the human frame, and in the cause and prevention of disease."
– Thomas Edison

Every parent wants to provide the best for their children. Most mothers watch what they eat and closely guard their health during pregnancy. But there's a secret I have found few people know before they start the adventure of parenthood.

The secret is both mother and father, upon receiving chiropractic care and removing toxins from their bodies, may improve their children's odds of lifelong good health before conception!

I stepped up my own chiropractic care when I discovered I was pregnant with my first child. I had a great pregnancy with no discomfort, pain or morning sickness. My daughter Morgan's delivery required no episiotomy. It was quick, easy and non-traumatic. Morgan weighed nine pounds, one-and-a half ounces. Not bad for a 5-foot, 2-inch, 110-pound woman!

After Morgan's birth, I fully understood the importance and scope of what chiropractic could do to prepare *both parents* before conception. In fact, what I learned was so profound I went back for specialized training and changed the focus of my practice from sports medicine to pregnancy and pediatrics!

In my opinion, it makes sense that a couple planning to become parents, who are taking care of themselves, could help their child achieve true wellness well before conception! In my practice, the first step is to help the couple get rid of toxins that may not allow their bodies to function at an optimum level by doing a specific whole body cleansing.

Every day, people breathe, eat and/or expose themselves to toxins. These toxins could cause problems with conception and a developing baby. I believe preparing the parents' bodies several months before conception could result in a better chance for a successful pregnancy and a healthy baby.

Nervous System Forms Within Days

It's common knowledge in child development circles that the brain and nervous system of the developing baby are in place within 21 to 28 days of conception. So before a woman may even know she's pregnant, the part of her baby's body that controls everything has already formed! This is why I believe preparing her body before conception is so critical.

In my practice, a very important part of this wellness protocol is for the couple to undergo several months of spinal adjustments before they plan to get pregnant. Restoring alignment to the spine may ensure the nervous system is functioning at peak levels to keep the body working at its best. Multiple case studies show chiropractic care can *help* couples conceive!

Could correcting and preventing subluxations be the key? Subluxations could result from injuries to the spine that could force the spinal bones out of alignment. Subluxations may occur due to a weakening of the spinal ligaments from chemicals or stress or a rip of the ligaments caused by trauma. The subluxation could pinch or irritate the spinal nerves that operate all physiological functions, making it harder for the organs to do their jobs.

Pain Is A Symptom Of A Process

It seems most people go to a chiropractor because of pain. What they may not understand is that pain may only be symptom of a degenerative process that could have started months, years or even decades before. Many times, symptoms could be due to multiple spinal injuries that may have compounded over the years.

Injured nerves could cause muscles to spasm, which may create inflammation. Inflammation could cause the body to produce scar tissue. This gum-like scar tissue glues the muscles together so they aren't able to perform properly. As a result, the muscles supporting the spine could even become permanently weak.

After a period of time, the inflammation could penetrate into the improperly moving joint complex, which is made up of tendons, ligaments, discs, nerves and bones. More scar tissue could form around the joint like an onion peel. By the time a patient goes to a chiropractor to alleviate pain, it could take more than just an adjustment or two to break down the scar tissue and repair the subluxation.

Babies And Moms Benefit From Chiropractic Care

Once a couple achieves pregnancy, chiropractic care could help the developing baby as much as the mother! In addition to keeping Mom comfortable during her pregnancy, keeping her as subluxation-free as possible could allow her nervous system to work correctly. This allows optimum blood flow and hormone function so the baby develops properly. In my practice, I believe it is important to keep the expectant mother as healthy as possible during her pregnancy with specific exercises, vitamins, diet, and most importantly, chiropractic care.

Procedures routinely performed in hospital deliveries often make labor longer and could affect the baby's health. Common practices like inducing labor by breaking the water, epidurals,

Caesarean sections, pulling the baby out with forceps or suction, or the common procedure of twisting and pulling on the baby's delicate head and neck with the doctor's hands could be very harmful. Dr. Abraham Towbin, M.D., a neuropathologist from Harvard Medical School, in the paper *Latent Spinal Cord and Brain Stem Injury in Newborn Infants,* found that subluxations do in fact occur during the birth process and can affect the baby's health.

Can Chiropractic Care Ease Delivery?

I believe and from my own experience, with regular chiropractic care, the length of labor may be cut by up to one-third and childbirth pain could be greatly diminished. According to Dr. Jeanne Ohm in her article *Chiropractic and Pregnancy: Greater Comfort and Safer Births* she states, "Chiropractic care throughout pregnancy can relieve and even prevent the common discomforts experienced during pregnancy."

She goes on to say about the birth, "Any baby position even slightly off during birth will slow down labor and add pain to both the mother and baby. Many women have been told that their babies were too big or labor 'just slowed down' when it was really the baby's presentation interfering with the normal process and progression."

By keeping the pelvis in correct alignment through chiropractic care, the baby has the room to grow and move. If the baby is in a breech or other abnormal position, there is a non-traumatic, specific adjustment called the Webster Technique that I can perform to get the baby to move into a head-down position.

I recommend the mother and father work with a midwife through the pregnancy and the delivery. They should be at home or in a warm, inviting birthing center for the birth. I believe the mother's emotional state is very important for both her and her baby. The sights, sounds and smells of a hospital could tend to make people experience a "fight or flight" response. This anxiety could affect the birth tremendously. I feel it could slow labor down, which could lead to more invasive procedures during delivery.

The births of my own children were stress-free and wonderful experiences. With my first child, I experienced only four hours of labor. I planned my second child and followed my pre-pregnancy protocol months before he was conceived. My pregnancy was how it should be — perfect. I worked up until the day I delivered and experienced virtually no labor at all! I was up walking around within hours of the birth and the next day I was already out at a restaurant.

Birth Could Cause Subluxations

I adjust newborns as soon as possible after birth because, even under the best circumstances, being born is traumatic and could cause subluxations. This is why I feel it is important for newborns to receive chiropractic care.

My staff and I teach new moms how to breastfeed and diaper their babies so they don't inadvertently cause subluxations. We also have important protocols as the baby grows to be a toddler, preschooler and all the way to adulthood to ensure good spinal hygiene.

Children Heal With Chiropractic Care

A number of my pediatric patients didn't have the benefit of their parents being at optimum health through chiropractic prior to or during pregnancy. Some of these children were delivered with forceps, Caesarean section or through induced labor and had very serious conditions. These conditions showed incredible improvement once the children received chiropractic treatment.

Dr. G. Gutmann, M.D., in his paper, *Blocked Atlantal Nerve Syndrome in Infants and Small Children*, reports that of more than 1,000 infants in the case study, approximately 80 percent or 800 had subluxations of the atlas from the birth process. The atlas is located where the skull and spinal column join. The study says that blocked atlas nerve impulses in infants develop conditions that range from central motor impairment and development, as well as, chronic childhood health problems like ear, nose and throat infections. These can be alleviated through chiropractic care. In the case study, Dr. Gutmann concluded that the 1,000 infants were treated successfully with chiropractic care almost without exception.

A 14-month-old named Megan was brought to me with chronic ear infections so bad she was on antibiotics perpetually for preventative measures. She had dark, sunken eyes and a pale face. After she underwent adjustments three times a week for a short period of time, the ear infections went away. She became a vibrant young child. Now she is a happy three-year-old and hasn't had a recurrence since!

A six-year-old with stage one scoliosis had a reversal after four months of chiropractic treatment. A breech baby whose mother underwent only three chiropractic adjustments turned head-down and was ready for delivery. Fourteen-month-old Mary has a tumor behind her eye and suffers anxiety at the doctor's office. After her first adjustment, she slept the entire night for the first time. She enjoys her chiropractic visits. An eight-year-old named Corey, who had always found it painful to walk and virtually impossible to run, can play with his friends now. The stories go on and on.

My goal as a Doctor of Chiropractic is to raise the babies of today to live long and healthy lives. I feel babies and their parents can achieve true wellness through chiropractic care. When people are well they seem to make better decisions, which may create healthier communities. The healthy babies of today will make a better world tomorrow.

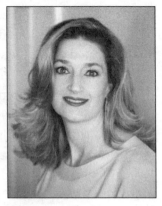

Dr. Claire H. O'Neill-Close, D.C., F.I.C.P.A
GlenFeliz Chiropractic Associates, Inc.
Los Angeles, California
(323)662-2891
www.drclaireoneill-close.com
www.glenfelizchiropracticassociates.com
Family wellness specializing in pregnancy
and pediatrics

Dr. Claire O'Neill-Close's experience in pharmacy altered her belief in true health from medicine to wellness, changing her life from medicine to chiropractic. Dr. Claire believes that true wellness can only be achieved by correcting and preventing subluxations. After Dr. O'Neill-Close's first child, she added pregnancy and pediatric care to her family and sports chiropractic practice. She attained her Fellowship in Pregnancy and Pediatrics from the International Chiropractic Pediatric Association.

The birth of her first child was a segment on *The Baby Story* for The Learning Channel (TLC). This showed the importance and benefits of chiropractic through her pregnancy and a natural water birth.

Dr. Claire O'Neill-Close is a sought-after expert who has been a regular guest on *Smart Solutions with Matty* on Home and Garden Television (HGTV). Dr. O'Neill-Close was published in the *Journal of the Neuromusculoskeletal System*, a chiropractic research journal. Dr. Claire has held many positions in various community, college and state associations. She is currently President of Alumni Association for Cleveland Chiropractic College, Los Angeles and has held this position for the past six years. Dr. Claire has received the Doctor of the Year Award by the California Chiropractic Association, San Fernando Valley district.

Dr. Claire provides care to families of all ages from pregnancy to the elderly, which focuses on the health of their spines to increase their optimal health and wellness.

Throughout her chiropractic career, she has discovered specific systems, behaviors and strategies that will significantly launch ordinary people to extraordinary health...youthful and energetic health through all ages.

If you would like to receive more information, schedule a private appointment with Dr. Claire or arrange for her to speak to your corporation or group call Dr. Claire's office at (323)-662-0733 or (323)-662-2891. You can also visit her web sites at www.glenfelizchiropracticassociates.com or www.drclaireoneill-close.com .

PART TWO

THE AMAZING SECRET THAT WILL IMPROVE YOUR HEALTH AND CHANGE YOUR LIFE

❧

Dr. Desirée Edlund, D.C., QME

You see them trudging to school with their heads slumped forward and their shoulders straining under the weight of bulging backpacks. Today's young people could be medical disasters in the making. Spinal damage could be inflicted early in life because of the combination of carrying heavy book bags, playing video games, sitting for hours at computers and various sports injuries.

Four out of five adults will develop back pain at some point in their life, as reported at www.mayoclinic.com/invoke.cfm?id=DS00171. Poor posture, starting as early as childhood, could be a major cause of this statistic.

Sometimes it takes a traumatic event to open our eyes to the importance of spinal health at a young age. In my case, I was 18 years old when a car accident changed my course in life. At the time, I was a pre-med major in college who was planning to become a plastic surgeon. After the accident, my days turned into nightmares. I was plagued by chronic headaches, pain in my upper back and neck and horrible posture.

I went to multiple doctors — a neurologist, an orthopedist and a general practitioner — looking for help. I even tried acupuncture, massage and physical therapy.

The doctors prescribed pain pills. I would treat my headaches with pain medication. Once the drugs wore off, my headaches came back.

Then the ugly cycle began. Headaches – Pills – More Headaches – More Pills. The use of Non-Steroidal Anti-Inflammatory Drugs (NSAIDs) including nonprescription aspirin puts over 107,000 patients in the hospital and kills between 12,840 and 16,050 residents of the U.S. every year! NSAIDs are medications which, as well as having pain-relieving effects, have the effect of reducing inflammation when used over a period of time.

A visit to the orthopedist was particularly traumatic for me. He threw my X-rays up on the light box, took a cursory glance, looked at me and said, "There's nothing we can do for you. You have to learn to live with the pain."

Live with the pain? At 18 years old, I could not comprehend dealing with chronic headaches and backaches for the rest of my life.

Upset, frustrated and desperate for relief from my pain, I searched for an answer.

That's when I turned to chiropractic care. My chiropractor addressed the misalignment in my neck. After several adjustments, the headaches and back pain were gone. What's more, my chiropractor also recognized my ongoing problem with poor posture. At 5 feet and 10 inches, I tended to slump to de-emphasize my height. By showing me how to correct my posture, my chiropractor helped prevent a lifetime of potential back pain.

After this life-changing experience, I decided to forego medical school and instead, I became a chiropractor. Today, I focus on helping patients of all ages head off potential health problems by ensuring they have good posture and healthy spines.

Your Child's Posture

Parents may choose to pay special attention to their children's spinal health starting at a young age. When children are around age six, parents should monitor children's postures to ensure they do not slouch, slump or hold their heads more forward than normal.

Poor posture could be the result of a number of seemingly harmless activities. These activities include playing video games and working on the computer. As children play computer games, they tend to sit on the floor and slump over without adequate support for their backs. This improper posture could train neck and back muscles to move out of a normal position. This could cause the bones of the spine to move into improper alignment. Sitting in front of a computer could have the same effect.

Today, we see more and more children hauling around huge backpacks that are one-third or more of their weight. Parents should be aware that overly stressing the back with a heavy backpack could cause back pain in their child. Over time, the damage could be significant and result in arthritis in the spine, neck and upper back.

Another source of spinal problems in children could be sports. These include high-contact sports like football, soccer, hockey or basketball. Other injury-causing activities include flexibility sports such as dance, gymnastics and cheerleading. Of course, participating in sports can be an important part of keeping kids active and healthy. But children who take part in these activities should have their spines checked throughout the growing years to be sure everything is aligned properly. Sports injuries may not be painful, or even noticed, when they occur. Instead, the injuries will most likely creep up on them later in life, which may result in chronic back and posture problems.

Good Posture

Heavy backpacks, poor posture and sports injuries may cause

misalignments of the spine. These misalignments, called subluxations, could suppress the energy flow of the body's nervous system. Over time this interruption of energy flow could cause an irritation to the spine and other organs of the body or nervous system. As a result, when children reach their twenties, thirties or forties, poor spinal health left untreated in childhood could come back to haunt them.

Teach children how to maintain good posture without slumping forward or holding their heads forward from their bodies while playing video games or working on the computer — even when wearing a backpack.

Many parents take their children to the pediatrician for a medical checkup each year. Include bringing children to a chiropractor for regular spinal checkups. This way a potential problem might be caught before it has the chance to become chronic or before permanent damage could take place.

In my office I check for subluxations using a computerized muscle and spine scan. This new technology could help detect early spinal problems and may illustrate any muscle imbalances your child may have. The test is painless and has no side effects.

If the spine is not properly aligned, the child may need a course of chiropractic adjustments designed to correct subluxations, increase the flow of energy throughout the body, and improve posture. I also put my patients on a posture correction program, utilizing a variety of rehab exercises and special types of traction.

Educating Patients

I help my patients with lifestyle changes to ensure ongoing spinal health. One of these changes involves backpacks, which I believe should not exceed ten to twenty percent of a child's body weight. Kids can also take advantage of ergonomic backpacks. These specialized packs use lumbar support to transfer the weight being carried from the upper back and neck to the lower portion of the spine. As a result, the child can stand up straight, and the weight load is decreased by about one-third. For kids who play video games, a floor pillow should be used to support the back and encourage good posture.

As children move into adulthood, they must continue to be aware of activities and habits that could compromise their posture and degrade their spinal health.

Adult Posture

Adults also must be wary of improper posture. Poor posture could lead to permanent, painful changes in the spine. The results could be aches, pains, numbness, tingling, headaches, internal organ problems or more.

Adults tend to develop posture problems while working on computers, experiencing repetitive stress and driving cars many miles a day. In each case, their bodies are contorted into unnatural positions.

When an adult patient comes to my office with posture difficulties, I first take a photo of the patient and use a computer program to evaluate his or her posture. Then the computer muscle and spine scan shows which muscles of the body are out of balance. Other tests include neurological/orthopedic exams and possibly an X-ray or MRI.

Typical treatments include spinal adjustments and different types of posture correcting traction. This is followed up by exercises to help strengthen the muscles and assist posture correction. After undergoing a course of treatment, a number of patients can see a dramatic difference in their posture and post treatment X-rays.

Ongoing care includes periodic adjustments of the spine, in addition to an awareness of habits and activities that can negatively influence spinal health. For example, I recommend patients who work on computers to take a break every 30 minutes. I instruct patients to sit up straight, and with their chins tucked in, to pull their heads and necks back over their shoulders and count to ten. Several repetitions of this may help prevent poor posture with the overall goal of maintaining good spinal health.

I also recommend a good lumbar support chair or a lumbar cushion placed in the small of the back while sitting. Good lumbar support is important for creating good posture while sitting.

The results of posture correction go beyond looking taller and more attractive. In my opinion, a patient who develops optimum posture could possibly live longer, have more energy, sleep better, be more flexible, have little or no pain and live a better quality of life. Posture correction with ongoing corrective care could have you reaping the benefits for a lifetime.

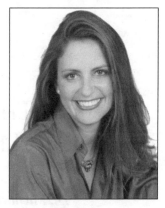

Dr. Desirée Edlund, D.C., QME
Essential Chiropractic
Irvine, California
949-724-0011
www.EssentialChiropractic.com

Dr. Edlund received her Doctorate degree with Magna Cum Laude honors from Southern California University of Health Sciences (formerly L.A.C.C.).

During her first few years of practice, Dr. Edlund moved to Minnesota and helped develop one of the first medical/chiropractic clinics in Minnesota, a state known for its medical establishments. She has worked hand-in-hand with established and reputable medical doctors.

Dr. Edlund started private practice in 1997 and currently is the Clinic Director and Founder of one of the fastest growing chiropractic clinics in Orange County, California.

Through her proven posture correcting rehab program, Dr. Edlund has successfully treated thousands of people who had been diagnosed with arthritis, fibromyalgia, headaches, chronic pain, carpal tunnel, allergies, acute injuries and TMJ (jaw problems).

She is happily fulfilling her purpose to help as many people as possible to obtain and maintain optimum levels of health and well-being. She practices what she preaches by getting adjusted weekly. This keeps her healthy and pain-free!

An avid spokesperson for the chiropractic profession, Dr. Edlund has made many television appearances on news programs and talk shows. She is also a prominent lecturer and co-author. Dr. Edlund is living her dream to educate the public about the science and miracles of chiropractic care.

To schedule a private appointment with Dr. Edlund or to arrange for Dr. Edlund to speak to your corporation or group, call 949-724-0011.

PART THREE

LIVING THE CHIROPRACTIC LIFESTYLE

❦

Dr. Michael McClellan, B.S., D.C.
Dr. Leslie McClellan, B.S., D.C.

My wife, Leslie, and I practice chiropractic as a profession and live what we call a chiropractic lifestyle.

What is the chiropractic lifestyle? We believe living a chiropractic lifestyle is a wholeness concept. First is recognizing the body as a completely integrated and functioning system. The brain sends continuous messages down the spinal cord and out the nerve roots to every single organ and cell in the body. We believe the body doesn't need a lot of help — it just doesn't need any interference.

A subluxation along the spine could block off or interfere with the central nervous system. It interrupts vital nerve flow to organs and cells in our bodies. Like a hose providing water to a flower, we cannot restrict this flow or the flower will die.

A study conducted in 1921 by Dr. Henry Windsor confirmed an almost 100 percent correlation between diseased organs and a misalignment or subluxation in the spine at the area related to that organ's nerve supply.

Dr. D.D. Palmer stated in 1895 that if the body could function as God planned it to function, it may never even develop a disease process.

Life Saving Adjustment

A beautiful and very special example was the birth of our son, Austin. He was a long and challenging home birth that labored on for 24 hours. When he finally appeared, he had swallowed meconium (a pre-birth bowel movement). This potential medical emergency could cause major respiratory problems, collapsed lungs and brain damage. Death is certainly a possibility.

Upon his arrival, the midwife tried to suction it out of him with a tube. I asked, "Did you get it all?" She said she didn't know. That was certainly not the answer I had hoped for.

Before fear could even begin to set in, something innate took over me. I asked my wife, Leslie, for our son. At five minutes old, I placed him on my arm and adjusted his spine. When I got to the upper thoracic area, he threw up the black tarry meconium and began to nurse.

Our son has never had a respiratory infection and at age six he has never had an antibiotic in his body.

Leslie and I have two children, both born at home. They receive regular adjustments and have perfectly aligned spines. By adjusting our children once a week, we know we are reducing the chance of health problems in our children.

How do we know? Neither of our children has ever taken an antibiotic. That doesn't mean our children have never gotten sick. However, part of the chiropractic lifestyle is realizing true wellness starts at birth. Our chiropractic lifestyle beliefs include that when a baby is born they are not born with a lack of anything. The human body is created with everything it needs to survive and heal itself.

Antibiotics are sometimes prescribed indiscriminately to children whose conditions don't warrant medication. This is possibly done just to ease parents' anxieties.

Moms and dads run to doctors when their children display the first sign of illnesses. Some parents seem to feel relief when doctors prescribe drugs to address illnesses.

However, Robert S. Mendelsohn, M.D., author of *How to Raise a Healthy Child in Spite of Your Doctor*, says parents can address most minor symptoms and illnesses without the use of drugs.

Do not misunderstand our view. We realize there are times in a child's life that require the attention of a medical doctor or pediatrician. However, for minor illnesses such as colds and low-grade fevers, we believe antibiotics are not the only answer.

Bodies Learning Wellness

If we continue to apply sickcare to our children, will their bodies learn wellnesscare? It's about wellness – proper diet, spinal care and avoiding drugs.

Accessmednet.com published a report on a study conducted by The World Health Organization, which concluded "about 14,000 people are infected and die each year as a result of drug-resistant microbes picked up in U.S. hospitals. More than 2 million Americans are infected each year and more than half of these infections resist at least one antibiotic."

The article continues, "Many medical researchers believe that a rapidly increasing resistance to antibiotics is one of the world's most pressing health problems."

In a study published in the *New England Journal of Medicine* conducted by the Active Bacterial Core Surveillance team — a program of the United States Centers for Disease Control and Prevention — researchers focused on bacteria that were increasingly resistant to multiple antibiotics. These included, but were not limited to, penicillin, cefotaxime, meropenem, erythromycin and trimethoprim-sulfamethoxazole. These resistant bacteria were found to be responsible for middle ear infection, pneumonia, meningitis and other common conditions.

Findings revealed 25 percent of the bacteria in the samples were resistant to penicillin. Resistance to at least three different types of antibiotics among patients jumped from 9 percent to 14 percent from 1995 to 1998.

Excess Medication

The U.S. Center for Disease Control and Prevention estimates that of the total 150 million prescriptions written for antibiotics each year in America, about 50 million are unnecessary.

Between human and animal use, America is using 30,000,000 pounds of antibiotics each year.

As parents, we realize how difficult it is to stand against the use of prescription drugs. When our son was four-years-old, his pre-school teacher told us he had ADD and needed to be medicated before he could start kindergarten.

This startled us in a number of ways. First, to have a kindergarten teacher telling us we needed to medicate our child in order for him to continue his education was alarming. As parents we felt our backs were against the wall.

However, we realized prescription drugs were not the answer. Proper nutrition and regular chiropractic care were our answers. I thought about all the parents who just went along with their educators and doctors needlessly medicating their kids.

It's interesting to watch our culture today. Antibiotics for sickness. Ritalin® (a class 2 narcotic) to start school. Anti-inflammatory medication, muscle relaxants and pain medication for sports. Then, children discover recreational drugs and parents freak out.

It's rather ironic we have a "Say No to Drugs" campaign, yet we put kids on prescription drugs, such as Ritalin®, before they are old enough to start kindergarten.

But no one has any idea of the long-term effects of these drugs. Jules Asher, a spokesman for the National Institute of Mental Health, was quoted in *USA Today* saying, "…no one knows what effect this stimulant has on children who take it for many years. Nor, (he says), does anyone know how the drug affects very young children."

That was certainly enough of a question for us to make a wiser health decision for our child. This helps us stay strong in our belief in the chiropractic lifestyle including proper nutrition, exercise on a regular basis and a strong faith in God.

We do believe the power that made our body is the only power that can truly heal this beautiful mechanism we call home. If we wear out our spine before we die, it will be a miserable place to live.

As family wellness providers, we encourage everyone to have a family chiropractic checkup. Chiropractic lifestyle and wellness apply to everyone. There are no age restrictions. We pray you will find chiropractic to be a major part of your life and wellness program.

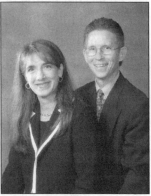

Dr. Michael McClellan, B.S., D.C.
Dr. Leslie McClellan, B.S., D.C.
McClellan Family Chiropractic Clinic
115 W. Grand Avenue, Suite 70
Rainbow City, Alabama 35906
(256)442-1441
mcchiro@internetpro.net

To schedule a private appointment with Dr. Michael or Dr. Leslie or to book either doctor to speak for your corporation or group, call (256) 442-1441.

PART FOUR

CHIROPRACTIC FOR CHILDREN: FINDING THE "FUN" IN PROPER FUNCTION

Dr. Will Hopson, D.C., and Dr. Lana Hopson, D.C.

Say the word "chiropractic" to the average person on the street and images of an adult seeking treatment for back pain will probably be the first thoughts springing to their minds.

Infants and children are almost never thought of as potential chiropractic patients. That's unfortunate. We believe chiropractic is an all-natural approach to achieving total wellness lasting your whole life — from conception to maturity. We feel its purpose is to uncover and eliminate all the barriers to our fullest health and growth potentials.

When you look at chiropractic as a broad-spectrum nurturing of mind and body, it suddenly becomes clear just how much children could gain from this special developmental support. Every child deserves the opportunity to thrive.

Common childhood disorders such as bed-wetting, sinus infections, ADHD, tonsillitis, colic and countless other miseries can take huge tolls on your child's self-esteem and day-to-day life.

As anyone who has ever parented an ailing child will tell you, poor pediatric health could also cause untold stress on the entire family. There aren't many situations more heartbreaking than watching your child sidelined, unable to fully participate in the pleasures of his or her once-in-a-lifetime childhood because of persistent illness. Unfortunately, it happens every day.

The good news is Pediatric Chiropractic care might help your children's wellness naturally, possibly quickly. We believe young bodies are designed to, at times, heal themselves.

If you're wondering how soon to start a child on a regimen of Pediatric Chiropractic care, the answer is simple…we recommend starting today. One might consider starting chiropractic care as early as the first day a mother learns she is expecting.

Pediatric Chiropractic For Pregnant Women

Most pregnant women wouldn't dream of missing even one dose of their daily pre-natal vitamins. At Hopson Chiropractic, we hope to make pre-natal chiropractic care as routine as taking vitamins. By seeing a chiropractor early and following through with regular visits, mothers-to-be might decrease the amount of trauma involved in the birth process for both herself and her child. How?

We believe it begins with a balanced maternal pelvis to allow additional mobility inside the womb. This could help the infant position in the best possible presentation for birth.

Dr. Jeanne Ohm, D.C., in her article, *Chiropractic Care in Pregnancy for Safer, Easier Births*, originally printed in International Chiropractic Pediatric Association Newsletter May/June 2001, reports on The Webster Technique which is a specific chiropractic adjustment for pregnant women discovered by Dr. Larry Webster. "Working to correct sacral subluxations, this technique balances pelvic muscles and ligaments in the woman's pelvis, removes constraint and allows the baby to get into the best possible position for birth. Results showed a high success rate in allowing babies in the breech position to go into the normal head down or vertex position. Because of its ability to facilitate easier, safer deliveries for both the mother and baby, many birth care providers are actively seeking Doctors of Chiropractic with the skills in this technique."

We believe the hands-on approach of chiropractic pre-natal care could also establish a bond between mothers and infants.

According to Michael Mendizza, in his article entitled *Bonding or Violence*, he writes about the research findings of Dr. James W. Prescott, Ph.D., Institute of Humanistic Science, "A baby's developing body and brain mirror and reflect, lifelong, the emotional-sensory environment provided by its first primary relationship, that is with its mother. The origins of love and violence take root in this first primary sensory environment. What we call 'affectional bonding' or nurturing, or its absence — very early in life — structures the developing brain to interpret the world and its relationships as peaceful, pleasurable and loving..."

Benefits For Infants And Older Children

Immediately after birth, we believe children could be checked for any of the possible adverse effects of the birthing process, such as torticollis or stress on the vertebrae. Torticollis is a condition in which the neck is twisted and the head inclined to one side.

As your child grows, countless falls become an inevitable part of the day as he or she learns to walk. Each bump on that diapered bottom could stress the spine. We believe it is crucial spinal alignment be maintained during this important time to ensure proper gait, posture and growth.

Reported at National Library of Medicine (www.ncbi.nlm.nih.gov) PubMed index number 2486187, according to *Infantile Colic Treated by Chiropractors: A Prospective Study of 316 Cases* by Klougart, Nilsson and Jacobsen from the Anglo-European College of Chiropractic, Bournemouth, England, "A prospective, uncontrolled study of 316 infants suffering from infantile colic and selected according to well-defined criteria shows a satisfactory result of spinal manipulative therapy in 94 percent of the cases. The median age of the infants was 5.7 weeks at the beginning of the treatment. The results were evaluated by analysis of a diary continuously kept by the mother and an assessment file comprised by interview. The study was carried out as a multi-center study lasting three months and involving 73 chiropractors in 50 clinics. The results occurred within two weeks and after an average of three treatments."

The Journal of Manipulative and Physiological Therapeutics, October 1999 published an article entitled *The Short-Term Effect of Spinal Manipulation in the Treatment of Infantile Colic: A Randomized Controlled Clinical Trial with a Blinded Observer*. It reported on infants, whose average ages ranged from 4.9 weeks to 5.9 weeks, who participated in a study showing the effects of spinal care versus medication in the treatment of infantile colic.

It was comprised of 50 infants whose parents consented to take part in the study. One group received spinal manipulation for two weeks; the other was treated with the drug dimethicone for two weeks. The results of the study were:

- By trial days four to seven, hours of crying were reduced by one hour in the dimethicone group compared with 2.4 hours reduced in the spinal manipulation group.
- On days eight through eleven, crying was reduced by one hour for the dimethicone group, whereas crying in the spinal manipulation group was reduced by 2.7 hours.
- From trial day five onward, the spinal manipulation group did significantly better than the dimethicone group.

The conclusion of the research study was a 67 percent reduction of the mean daily hours with colic on day twelve for the infants receiving spinal care. The dimethicone group only had a reduction in daily hours with colic of 38 percent by day twelve. The study concluded that spinal manipulation is effective in relieving infantile colic.

As Donald Epstein, D.C. says in his article, *Healthy Children and Chiropractic,* originally printed in the *International Chiropractic Pediatric Association Newsletter* of January/February 1998, "In the course of chiropractic care, it is common for parents to remark that their child's disposition has improved, that he learns better in school, that she is more at peace, that he reacts to stress more effectively, sleeps better, and that in general he is more able to function without restriction. These are all indicators of health."

With Pediatric Chiropractic, we believe you'll be giving your children a gift far greater than any video game system or shiny, new mountain bike. You could be offering them a chance at longevity and endurance, optimal health and the prevention of some diseases.

Plus, chiropractic care is a drug-free, natural wellness lifestyle. By starting early, your kids could develop good health habits to see them through their entire lifetimes. Practices like proper nutrition, adequate rest, ample hydration and spinal alignment could ensure your family members enjoy the vitality they deserve.

To learn more about Pediatric Chiropractic, visit the website for the International Chiropractic Pediatric Association at www.icpa4kids.com. There you'll read about the benefits of proper spinal alignment for children of all ages. You will discover where to attend seminars in your area and even get help locating a nearby chiropractic pediatric practitioner. Or, stop by www.chiropediatrics.com to learn when the next free Pediatric Chiropractic screening for Kids Day International will be available in your area.

Childhood should be a time of laughter, learning, love and achievement. Help your child discover how "fun" health and wellness can truly be. Call for your Pre-Natal or Pediatric Chiropractic exam today.

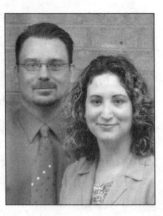

Dr. Will Hopson, D.C.
Dr. Lana Hopson, D.C.
Hopson Chiropractic
4411 Old Bullard Rd. Ste 500
Tyler, Texas 75703
Phone (903) 581-4393
Fax (903) 581-8511

To schedule a private appointment with Dr. Will or Dr. Lana or to book either doctor to speak for your corporation or group, call (903) 581-4393.

CHAPTER FOUR

HEALTH SECRET HELPS REAL LIFE PEOPLE

PART ONE

MANY PEOPLE JOINING THE WELLNESS CLUB

Dr. Lynne Sullivan D.C.

As a student athlete at University of California Davis, I was always interested in health sciences.

While playing basketball, I injured my back. I went to the school clinic where I was given painkillers and muscle relaxants. When this didn't work, I tried physical therapy. The therapy and massage felt good, but the pain would return after a few days. I still couldn't play.

It was suggested I give up sports. At the age of 21, the thought was unacceptable. A friend recommended I try chiropractic care. I was desperate enough to try anything!

I was amazed. Within a few weeks, I was feeling great and back on the court. I became fascinated by the profession and decided to become a chiropractor. I graduated from chiropractic college in 1986 and have been in private practice ever since.

The Wellness Connection

During my career as a chiropractor, I have found people do not understand the link between chiropractic care and wellness.

Most people judge their health based on how they feel. When they feel ill they go to see their medical doctor and might take pills for relief. But, I believe, pills cannot provide true wellness.

How does the pill know what organ to go to? Or how much of a certain chemical your body needs exactly where?

Healing From Within

I believe true health really comes from within. And the power that made the body has the power to heal the body. By removing subluxations, chiropractors could open channels to true health. This may give bodies options to heal without drugs or surgeries.

When patients come into my office, very few are aware of how to achieve true wellness. Most seek chiropractic care as last resorts after trying physical therapies, a variety of medicines or surgeries.

Our new patients are usually referred from our current patients who have achieved improved health and are excited about the results from our office.

We were taking care of a young woman who was injured in an automobile accident. During the course of her care, the irritable bowel syndrome she had battled for years cleared up! She was so excited. On a subsequent visit to her medical doctor, she told her story. The doctor was intrigued. He gave me a call for lunch.

After our lunch meeting, he asked if I would help him with wellness. He didn't really have any specific health complaints, but he wanted to see if chiropractic would improve his overall state of health.

He has completed his initial care and is the first medical doctor in our Wellness Club program. He reports feeling much better overall and regularly refers patients to our office. He stated his patients who are under chiropractic care are seen less often in his office than those who are not under chiropractic care. Wellness works!

One of the reasons I enjoy being a chiropractor is I don't have to put anything into the body. I don't have to take anything out. Chiropractic care allows people to heal inside out, naturally. Chiropractic care offers a person the ability to achieve his or her own individual level of wellness.

Our office specializes in wellnesscare. It is my hope patients will see value and incorporate chiropractic care in their arsenal of good health habits. We care for newborns all the way through senior citizens. Our office is truly a family practice.

Help For Ear Infections

I have noticed ear infections, unfortunately, have become common in young people. We had a mom bring in her 3-year-old son who suffered from ear infections most of his life. He had taken many forms of antibiotics to no avail. His parents had tried everything and were quite distraught. It was suggested that he have surgery to place tubes in his ears. It can be very frightening and frustrating when nothing seems to help your sick child.

The results for this boy were wonderful. After just 3 adjustments, the ear infection was gone. To this day, he is ear infection free! No miracles. Just proper nerve function.

Another Option

Another female patient of mine was what I call a hit-or-miss patient. She wasn't good at keeping her appointments. We typically only saw her when she had symptoms.

Her excuse was she was to too busy as a real estate professional. I hear this excuse often. Unfortunately, people don't realize how valuable their health is until they no longer have it.

One day she called me from the hospital and told me doctors were going to amputate her arm. She said about a week earlier she had a severe neck pain. Her arm began to swell. The doctors told her she had a serious infection in her arm and it could not be brought under control through antibiotics. She was told if they didn't amputate her arm, she might die.

The patient told me she firmly believed whatever was afflicting her arm had something to do with her neck. She asked me to see her in the hospital and give her an adjustment. I did.

The next day I stopped back at the hospital and noticed her arm swelling went down 50 percent. The doctors said it was a miracle. I had simply freed the entrapped nerve, allowing it to resume function.

I adjusted her again at the hospital. She was released a couple days later, pain and infection free, with her arm still attached. She was so excited. She introduced me to all her floor mates and healthcare providers.

Safe Chiropractic

One of the reasons I commonly hear for not seeing a chiropractor is that adjustments hurt or a person might be harmed in some way. In the past 18 years as a chiropractor, I have given over 216,000 adjustments and have no malpractice claims for injury. I'm sure most of my colleagues can report a similar success rate. In my experience, chiropractic is safe and effective.

I see one of my main functions as a chiropractor is to accept patients at their individual levels of health understanding. Over time, I help them increase their knowledge of how to achieve true health.

To me, the word "doctor" actually means "teacher." I see this as the most challenging role. When patients first enter my office they typically come for a specific health concern and usually after all other methods have failed. It is exciting to me to when chiropractic care improves multiple aspects of their health and wellbeing, more than just their neck and back pains.

As a society, we typically look for "quick fixes." Chiropractic care is not a quick fix. Realizing a health condition may have been deteriorating for years, it is sensible to believe a turnaround may take some time.

In my experience, many patients make the switch from pain management to wellnesscare in about six months. Although most patients report feeling better within the first few weeks of care,

I have found, it takes an ongoing program of wellnesscare to truly stabilize the spine and allow the body to heal itself.

Our Wellness Club members realize how chiropractic care can enhance their overall health and wellness. For example, my son is now 16 and has missed only one day of school due to illness. He has been adjusted since birth.

In my 18 years of practice, I have only missed one day due to illness. I've received chiropractic care once per week since I was 21.

Drug Jug

Perhaps my favorite thing in the office is a big jar called the Drug Jug. As their medical doctors are allowing my patients to go off medication, my patients happily throw their drugs into the Drug Jug. It is exciting to see increasingly more patients throwing their drugs in the Drug Jug.

One lady threw away five different types of medications after being on them for a work-related injury seven years prior. No miracles, just good chiropractic care!

In my opinion, if the general public truly understood chiropractic and its benefits, all chiropractors would have lines of patients waiting to be adjusted.

If I had one wish as a chiropractor, it would be for everyone to enjoy the wonderful health benefits chiropractic offers from the cradle to the grave. I believe we would be a healthier, happier nation.

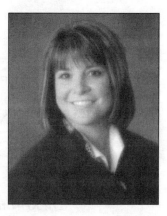

Dr. Lynne Sullivan, D.C.
Sullivan Chiropractic Health Center
268 Main Street
Pleasanton, California 94566
(925) 484-1070
www.drsully.com
Specializing in wellnesscare

Dr. Lynne Sullivan graduated as the class valedictorian from Life Chiropractic College-West in 1983. In a short period of time, she built a very busy family practice specializing in wellnesscare. The readers of her local California paper have voted her office "Best" for a decade.

Dr. Sullivan provides care to the spine and nervous system, which helps restore optimal health. Through her 18 years as a practicing chiropractor, she discovered specific systems that launch ordinary people to extraordinary health...youthful and energetic health at most any age. Using her special technique, she has helped thousands of patients achieve great results where other methods have fallen short or failed.

Dr. Sullivan is a sought-after expert, speaker and media guest. She has been a college instructor and authored many published articles. Dr. Sullivan's work has been featured in numerous media including newspaper, magazines and TV.

To schedule a private appointment with Dr. Sullivan, find out more about the Wellness Club or to arrange for Dr. Sullivan to speak to your corporation or group, call (925) 484-1070.

PART TWO

LIVE LONGER LIVING OR LIVE LONGER DYING?

∽

Dr. Kristin M. Kidgell, B.S., D.C.

What if I said to be as healthy as possible you have to think like a child?

My six-year-old son, Nicholas, always asks the question, "Why?" If you have ever been around children, you know exactly what I'm talking about. Until they are satisfied and understand the information, children repeatedly ask the question, "But why?"

However, when it comes to their health, adults have stopped asking, "Why?" This is a serious issue! In a moment, I will tell you about a patient who started asking "why" and how that one word changed his life from a downward spiral to an uplifting future.

I truly believe my patients of all ages live their lives to the fullest potential because I take the time to educate each patient. I review how the body is created to work and explain why it does what it does. This review sparks patients to ask "why" to everything they encounter and ultimately enables them to enhance their health and lives.

Why would you bother learning more about yourself? Why settle for anything less than the best you can be?

Opinions Are Like Noses…Everyone Has One!

Don't make healthcare decisions based on someone else's opinion. Decide for yourself by asking questions until you completely understand the answers. It's your health, so take control of it! Then *you, too,* could make better decisions and live longer living instead of live longer dying!

The first thing I want to make clear is the definition of health. If you want to achieve optimal health, you must understand its true meaning. So, how do most people define health? I ask that question to groups of people every week and get the same answer. Basically, they believe that health is defined by how they feel. For example, they say, "I'm healthy if I feel good."

So if you feel poorly you must be sick? Are you ready for the shocker? In my opinion, this way of "symptom thinking" is absolutely the wrong way to judge your health. If you keep doing what your neighbors, loved ones and co-workers are doing, you could end up like others, suffering needlessly, either now or later.

Waiting for symptoms is the same as ignoring your health. Ignoring your health could cause it to deteriorate. You must attempt to maintain your good health everyday. This is most often referred to as prevention.

Ask yourself what type of quality of life do you want to have in 10 or 20 years.

Dorland's Medical Dictionary (twenty-fifth Ed.) states the definition of health is "a state of optimal physical, mental, and social well-being, and not merely the absence of disease and infirmity."

Simply put, health is how well your body is *functioning*, not merely the absence of symptoms. Confused? Stick with me.

Let's say I share a hamburger with someone and, unknowingly, the meat is bad. A while later, I'm in the bathroom vomiting from the meat. Yet the other person feels fine. My question is why did only I get sick? Clearly, the bad meat made me sick.

Whose body is working better? Is it mine throwing up the bad meat or the other person's keeping in the toxic food?

The other person's body is not functioning optimally. In this example, symptoms do not necessarily mean there is something going wrong in the body, and a lack of symptoms does not mean the other person is healthy. (You may want to reread that last sentence until you say "AH-HA.")

Here's another! The first symptoms of a heart attack are chest pain and shortness of breath. These symptoms are the last thing to show up, though the disease has been in motion for years. What about cancer? By the time you start feeling poorly (symptoms) from cancer it may have already spread into its deadly phases.

Is this starting to make sense? Can you see how symptoms could be misleading?

Let's say you have been unintentionally ignoring your health and it is starting to "talk" to you by possibly giving you symptoms. Even when symptoms surface, most people never ask why the symptoms appear. They either ignore them hoping they will go away or they take some sort of medication they hope will alleviate the symptoms. Fever — medicine, headache — medicine, diarrhea — medicine, ear infection — medicine, arthritis — medicine.

When did we stop asking *why do I have a fever? Why do I keep getting headaches? Why do kids get ear infections or asthma?*

The first step is to ask why. I believe this is your best chance to live healthier and to your best potential. Understanding how and why the body works the way it does could allow you to ultimately make better choices and extend your life.

A Cause Instead of A Label

Authors have written many books about the body's ability to fight germs and heal itself. Some have said doctors should be concentrating on prevention and *stimulating* the body's natural healing powers. These books show how some medications prevent a disease from expressing itself symptomatically while the disease progressively worsens.

So the next step is to ask the question, "What do I do?"

You need to make sure your body is functioning properly without anything holding it back. Basically, give yourself a chance! As you know, good function allows for good health and bad function allows for dis-ease.

So, what controls *all* of the body's functions? The brain and the nervous system.

Do you remember what happened to Christopher Reeve, the actor who played Superman? He fell off a horse and broke two bones in his neck, sliced his spinal cord and was left paralyzed from the neck down. Many of his brain's "life messages" can no longer reach his organs, limbs and immune system.

When these inborn, innate messages are stopped or slowed, this state could ultimately stop or slow proper functioning and healing to the areas of the body needing that full nerve supply.

Let's change the scenario. Instead of cutting or tearing the spinal cord, let's just compress it. Squeeze it, choke it or pinch it. This is what a subluxation does.

For example, if someone has a subluxation that chokes the "life messages" to his or her lungs, ears, intestines, kidney or stomach, these body parts could start to *malfunction*. Over time, this could lead to dis-ease. It is then possible maladies such as asthma, ear infections, constipation or diarrhea, acid reflux or ulcers may develop later.

You could take a medication to work on the symptoms or you could recognize the malfunction by asking the question, why. "Why is my stomach having these problems?" Then take aim to work on the cause. Could it be due to lack of nerve messages because of pressure on the nerves? Sounds complicated, but it really isn't. It is simple anatomy and physiology.

Research is becoming more and more prevalent today. For

example, according to a study conducted by Dr. Pikalov, M.D., Ph.D., entitled *Use of Spinal Manipulation Therapy in the Treatment of Duodenal Ulcer: A Pilot Study* published in the *Journal of Manipulative Physiological Therapeutics* it reported, "The use of spinal manipulative therapy resulted in pain relief from ulcers after one to nine days (average of 3.8 days) and clinical remission an average of 10 days earlier than traditional care."

What Is This "S" Word?

It is pronounced "sub-lux-ay-shun." Although, I am thrilled when patients call it the "S" word!

Subluxations can occur at any level of the spine and could cause multiple malfunctions. These obstructions to your nervous system could compromise your body's ability to function and heal properly.

For example, a subluxation can cause the head and neck to shift forward. This forward head posture or position will not only make your body hunch, but could eventually cause dis-ease.

If your spine is deteriorating, the spinal cord could also be deteriorating and not sending the messages out! Left unidentified and uncorrected, it could worsen and possibly become permanent.

Doctors of Chiropractic are the only wellness doctors trained to identify and remove subluxations. X-rays can show subluxations of the spine. A picture is worth a thousand words.

Thinking you are healthy because you don't have symptoms is misleading and could be deadly. I recommend the first wellness step is to find out if you have subluxations that can be fixed. The removal of subluxations could allow your body to function and heal the best it possibly can to prevent dis-ease. This could, in turn, allow you to live longer living instead of live longer dying.

All Hope Is *Not* Lost

Other chapters in this book are filled with stories about children and adults who have had the most amazing experiences with their chiropractic care. I, too, am going to share a patient's story. I have yet to see anyone come through my doors in worse shape. So this should give anyone hope, which I feel is the one thing most people are not given anymore. When you read his story, ask yourself was he living longer *living* or was he living longer *dying* on that first visit?

Richard, a 67-year-old patient, had seen many specialists for multiple health conditions before he first came to see me. His various doctors had him on a whopping 24 different medications. Richard hardly walked outside, went to the store or traveled to see his grandchildren.

Richard came in with his wife to see if chiropractic care could help him walk without pain or his cane. He had just ordered a wheelchair and was not looking forward to using it. After they attended my *New Patient Orientation*, he started asking, "Why?" Richard decided to not just focus on pain, but to work on enhancing the function of his entire body.

I was nervous adjusting Richard for the first time because there was so much wrong with him. But when Richard walked in to his next visit without his cane, our entire office was excited.

Every week Richard came in with more and more exciting news about how his health was returning. In three months, his doctors cut his medications almost in half! Richard followed my care plan and in approximately 10 months he went from four leaky heart valves to one. He avoided kidney surgery and doesn't use his breathing medications anymore.

Now Richard and his wife come in every month to maintain all they have accomplished. His doctors continue to reduce his medications!

Richard once told me he didn't even think he would see his 70th birthday. Well, that birthday has come and gone and he now enjoys long walks and vacations to see his great-grandchildren 4,000 miles up north.

Richard was right on when he said, "I thank God for giving Dr. Kidgell the knowledge and the hands to make the corrections for my body to self-heal."

Life Is A Gift

For generations our society has been brought up in houses with built-in medicine cabinets. It is no wonder we think and act the way we do. Dr. Barbara Starfield, M.D. wrote an article for *The Journal of the American Medical Association*, July 26, 2000,Volume 284, ranking the United States *second to last* in overall health compared to other countries. Of 13 countries in a recent comparison, the United States ranked an average of 12th. Countries in order of their ranking on health indicators, starting with the top ranked country in the world and ending with the lowest ranking health performance were Japan, Sweden, Canada, France, Australia, Spain, Finland, Netherlands, United Kingdom, Denmark, Belgium, United States and Germany.

The World Health Organization confirmed this poor performance by the United States with their own independent health system study which ranked the U.S. 15th out of 25 industrialized countries.

The United States' perception of the rankings is that the American's smoking, drinking and carrying out violence explains the poor ranking.

The statistics show otherwise. In the United States, 24 percent of females and 26 percent of males smoke. In Denmark (ranked better than the United States), 41 percent of females smoke. In Japan (ranked number one), 61 percent of males smoke.

Both Denmark and Japan have more smokers, yet better health results for their people than we have here in the United States.

Alcohol, violence and diet are comparatively the same. The United States ranks as having lower alcohol consumption, less violence and better diet than many other countries in the study. Yet the U.S. still ranks, worldwide, as having the second worst health results.

And, too, a little more than 100 years ago, the use of leeches for blood letting was the main medical treatment for ailments. The time has come to put away the myths and misunderstandings!

Chiropractic is not a treatment for a disease or a symptom. Chiropractic is the only healthcare system focusing on the spine for nervous system interference caused by subluxations. Specific adjustments remove nerve pressure and allow inborn, God-given potential to be expressed with the goal of optimal healing and function.

I urge you to cherish the life you have been given. Choose wisely how you take care of it. I encourage you to get regular spinal subluxation check ups for you and your children to help ensure a healthier tomorrow.

"Do not conform any longer to the pattern of this world,
but be transformed by the renewing of your mind."
– Romans 12:2

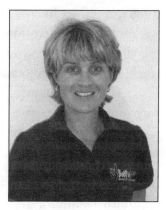

Dr. Kristin M. Kidgell, B.S., D.C.
Advanced Chiropractic
Bradenton, Florida
(941)752-3352

Dr. Kidgell is an expert in gentle and precise wellnesscare for the entire family. She specializes in Pediatric Chiropractic Care and Rehabilitative Corrective Care for all ages.

To schedule a private appointment with Dr. Kidgell or to arrange for Dr. Kidgell to speak to your school, corporation or group, call (941)752-3352.

PART THREE

Achieving Optimum Wellness Leads To Longer, Healthier Lives

By Dr. William J. Brady, D.C

More and more Americans are reaching retirement age and have begun experiencing the aches and pains that go along with it! Little do they know that chiropractic care could not only eliminate their stiffness and soreness, but it also might help them lead longer, healthier lives.

As a third-generation chiropractor, I've witnessed the healing abilities of the body. I watched my grandfather practice. My uncle took up his profession. Today, in my 14th year of practice, I offer patients a natural way to encourage their bodies to perform at their best.

Many of my patients are senior citizens. They come to me experiencing low back pain, neck pain, knee problems and other symptoms of aging. One of the biggest problems my patients face is fear of growing older. It's amazing to see when their aches and pains go away through chiropractic care how they can enjoy the little things in life again, like walking and exercising.

I spend a lot of time with my patients explaining chiropractic and helping to ease their fears that chiropractic adjustments might hurt.

I explain to them there is a wide variety of chiropractic adjusting techniques, including gentle ones for delicate bones. Their fears subside. After they have their first chiropractic adjustment, they can't wait for the next one!

I also work with my patients to take up exercise programs and begin following healthy diets. I frequently recommend supplements so their bodies will function at the optimum levels for good health.

Our younger and middle-aged patients benefit from chiropractic as well. They go on and on about how their headaches went away or how after struggling for years with neck and low back pain that they were able to get some relief with chiropractic adjustments.

My patients often still see medical doctors, and I work hand in hand with the patient's medical practitioners. Physicians in my community refer patients to me. At times, I refer patients to physicians as well.

Focus On Wellness

One of the most common misconceptions about chiropractic is you are "cured" after just a few adjustments. Most people will give pills 30 chances to work. What a number of patients have found is that if they give half as many adjustments a chance, they'll be amazed at the difference!

Medical doctors usually are focused on disease, while chiropractors tend to be focused on obtaining total wellness. We do this by harnessing the body's ability to heal itself with its innate healing forces. There are some diseases that can't be cured. In those situations, chiropractic could give a patient a better quality of life by ensuring maximum nerve flow to all parts of the body.

Wellness could be hindered by subluxations, or misaligned vertebrae of the spine, which interfere with the nervous system's ability to function normally. These subluxations could be caused by diet, lack of exercise, stress, pollution or injury. I believe it's virtually impossible today to avoid subluxations.

We try to make our office a stress-free retreat for our patients. My friendly staff creates a "wow" experience that includes massage therapy, personal nutritional counseling, hydrotherapy and chiropractic care. Our patients can attend yoga and tae kwon do classes or work with a personal fitness trainer. Patients also have access to information about diets and supplements, something I consider very important to overall health.

New patients to my office first are examined, X-rayed if necessary, and treated with appropriate therapies and a hydro massage. We give them a report of findings and begin their chiropractic care.

We also go over their lifestyle choices. It's important for patients to give up their bad habits to allow the innate healing force of their bodies to work. Diet is a big issue — people can put a lot of toxins in their bodies. We encourage patients to eat more whole grains, fruits and vegetables. We also suggest good multivitamins and nutritional supplements for optimum health.

Physicians in my community refer obstetrics patients to my clinic. It is my experience that mothers-to-be could be a lot more comfortable during pregnancy and deliver much faster and easier if they are subluxation-free.

Several of the gentle care techniques I use for pregnant women are also commonly used with my senior patients. Pelvic blocking techniques use the weight of the body to move the sacrum and pelvis to fix subluxations. There's no manual adjusting involved – just the weight of the body moving the spine. We also focus on trigger point manipulation for our more delicate patients.

I see children in my practice. I usually have to tell their parents I won't adjust their little ones the same way I adjust a young adult. There are a wide variety of chiropractic techniques that are safe and effective for the 9-day-old baby, 9 months pregnant mother-to-be and 90-year-old woman!

Another gentle treatment method involves a small adjusting tool. By using this tool, we can achieve the same results without putting any force on the patient. I use it often with children and elderly people with delicate bones.

Through chiropractic adjustments, my patients begin feeling better. They may find chiropractic corrects more than aches and pains. It can change lives.

Rewards Of Chiropractic

It's rewarding to see how chiropractic can benefit others. My office receives a number of thank-you notes and testimonials every week. Here are just some of their stories:

One patient, whose husband had been under chiropractic care for some time, came in after years of suffering from back pain. She was thrilled to finally get some relief. She really believed that's all chiropractic was about.

This patient and her husband had been trying for five years to have a second child. Her first pregnancies were very difficult. She suffered two miscarriages. As she continued her chiropractic care, she discovered she was pregnant. Her pregnancy was easy, and she gave birth to a healthy baby.

A 63-year-old patient has avoided cortisone treatments in her arthritic knee with help from chiropractic care.

An elderly patient with leg and back pain reports she has been able to walk without a cane after receiving chiropractic care.

The mother of a young cheerleader reports that her daughter's aches and pains have gone away, and she no longer gets colds when the weather changes. All since she began chiropractic care.

I'm proud of these success stories and the hundreds of others that occur every year in my office. People in my community are discovering they can live fuller, more productive, pain-free lives with regular chiropractic care.

I have files and files of letters from patients just like these telling me how chiropractic care has helped them resume normal lives. My 18-year-old daughter has seen the transformation that occurs when people achieve wellness. She works in my office now, and both she and her 12-year-old brother are interested in becoming chiropractors. I'm proud that there may be a fourth-generation chiropractor in the Brady family. I'm certain they will continue the legacy of helping people achieve wellness by empowering people to let their bodies heal themselves.

Dr. William J. Brady, D.C.
LifeCare Chiropractic Clinic
406 Pte Tremble
Algonac, Michigan 48001
(810) 794-5000
Drbill4042@aol.com
www.lifecarechiroclinic.com

As a graduate from Life College of Chiropractic, Dr. Brady has practiced family chiropractic care for 14 years at his office, LifeCare Chiropractic Clinic. Dr. Brady has discovered specific chiropractic care which could help you feel younger and more energetic. He speaks to organizations and is a radio and television guest. Dr. Brady's goal is to make his community a healthier place one spine at a time.

To schedule an appointment with Dr. Brady or to arrange for Dr. Brady to speak to your corporation or group, call (810) 794-5000.

PART FOUR

CHIROPRACTIC CARE FOR ADDICTIONS AND NEUROLOGICAL PROBLEMS

～⁂～

Dr. Brian Stearns, D.C., C.Ad.

When someone sustains whiplash in a rear-end collision or a severe sprain during a touch-football game, he or she may turn to a chiropractor for help. In fact, a number of patients choose a chiropractor to treat their aches and pains.

Chiropractors could also provide a haven for patients suffering from some forms of internal disorders and neurological deficits. Some patients may have been failed by other medical choices and continue to live with the debilitating effects of everything from cerebral palsy to autism to addictions.

Neurological problems are not traditionally thought of as candidates for chiropractic care. But in some cases, chiropractic care may offer the only hope for improvement.

Health Turning Point

A dramatic example of this is Tabby, a patient I first saw when she was 14 years old. Since birth, Tabby had suffered from a host of neurological problems. She was born prematurely and weighed only one pound, nine ounces. In fact, in the delivery room, Tabby was considered stillborn and placed to the side while the doctors attended her mother. Only a tiny whimper indicated she was alive at all.

When the doctors heard her distress, they resuscitated Tabby and placed her in an incubator. As a result of this exposure, Tabby became blind and suffered mental developmental problems. Other early difficulties included scoliosis, which forced her to wear braces on her lower legs.

As a small child, Tabby was given immunizations that caused an allergic reaction, ultimately producing diagnoses of autism and epilepsy.

Tabby was frightened and recoiled at the slightest touch when her parents first brought her to my office. We allowed her to gradually become accustomed to the office. At first, she simply came into the office and sat in the reception area where she could become used to the sounds, smells and people around her. Gradually, she entered other rooms. Eventually she was comfortable coming into the examination room for testing.

After performing a battery of tests and examining her X-rays, I determined Tabby had several subluxations, or interferences in the nervous system.

Over four months, I performed adjustments to Tabby's spine to alleviate the subluxations. This retrained her nervous system, enabling it to work more efficiently

Almost immediately, Tabby began showing signs of improvement. Her parents said she appeared more mentally sharp than ever before. She grew more inquisitive, asking questions about the things she heard around her.

Tabby gained a newfound freedom. One day she was at the hospital for an evaluation. Those attending her left her at the elevator, explaining she should push the button to go up. They told Tabby they would meet her upstairs. To everyone's excitement, Tabby was able to follow their directions and take the elevator on her own.

Tabby continues to enjoy improvement. Today, she no longer needs body or leg braces. She can get up and walk across a room on her own, something she could not easily perform previously. And to the joy of her father, Tabby is more communicative than ever before. She is even reading and writing in Braille. Tabby's father says the turning point was chiropractic treatment.

For patients like Tabby, a chiropractor can perform several diagnostic tests not offered by traditional medical doctors. One of these is thermography, which measures temperatures on the surface of the body. The thermograph can detect variances in body temperature on the skin, which may correlate to problems in the patient's autonomic nervous system.

Another important test is surface electromyography. This measures the muscle activity in the body to determine whether muscles are working too hard, or not hard enough. It shows whether muscles are working together or if one side of the body is working harder than the other side.

These two tests together can reveal some of the workings of the nervous system, including any abnormal neurological patterns generated by subluxations.

Subluxations can be caused by three sources: physical injuries; chemical influences including poor diet or being exposed to certain chemicals, drugs and alcohol; and most importantly, emotional distress.

When subluxations occur, they could suppress the energy flow of the body's nervous system. These are essentially neurological deficits, which could affect various cell tissues and organs.

Addictions

I believe a large percentage of the population has a neurological and/or genetic predisposition to addictive behaviors. These behaviors can fall into five categories: drugs and alcohol, food, sex, work and risk taking or gambling. With these and other compulsive conditions, I feel the nervous system essentially gets stuck in a rut. Any time patients experience stressful situations, they respond in the same ways. They may eat, drink or gamble excessively. They may choose other obsessive or harmful behaviors.

Why does this happen? There is a series of chemical events in the brain called the Brain Reward Cascade.

It has been studied by the Department of Biological Sciences at the University of North Texas and others. The studies concluded brains with compromised dopamine D2 receptors cause individuals to "have a high risk for multiple addictive, impulsive and compulsive behaviors such as severe alcoholism, cocaine, heroin, marijuana and nicotine use; glucose bingeing, pathological gambling, sex addiction, ADHD, Tourette's Syndrome, autism, chronic violence, post-traumatic stress disorder, schizoid/avoidant cluster, conduct disorder and antisocial behavior."

The report states dopamine is released in the brain and stimulates dopamine receptors. Dopamine is referred to as the "pleasure molecule" and the "antistress molecule."

The report concludes that when the Brain Reward Cascade is not functioning well, a person may require dopamine "fixes" to feel good. Alcohol, cocaine, heroin, marijuana, nicotine and glucose all cause activation and neuronal release of brain dopamine, which could satisfy abnormal cravings.

Unfortunately, many people afflicted by these addictive behaviors find little relief. If they visit a doctor and ask for assistance, they likely will be offered drugs. But I believe that the practice of prescribing drugs to people with already addictive personalities is playing with fire. That's why I promote chiropractic care as a promising choice for addicts, since chiropractic care is drug-free.

Healing Addiction

When helping an addictive patient, I care for the whole person. My program is specifically geared toward alleviating the symptoms of withdrawal, diminishing cravings and helping the body break its chemical predisposition to addiction with the goal of the body healing itself.

First, I determine whether the patient really wants to stop the addictive behavior. This is absolutely necessary for success. As a chiropractor, I cannot take more responsibility for the patient's health than they are willing to take themselves.

If the addiction is severe, I refer the patient to counseling as an important part of his or her care program. This could include one-on-one therapy or group treatment in a setting such as Alcoholics Anonymous, or a combination of these.

Next are chiropractic adjustments, which are designed to remove subluxations and increase the flow of energy throughout the body. Once this flow is restored, the body may unleash its own healing power known as innate intelligence.

With the nervous system working properly, the body may have an intrinsic ability to heal itself. In the case of addictive behavior, as in any other health challenge, unlocking the body's innate intelligence could assist the individual in reaching his or her optimal genetic and spiritual potential.

Another effective technique is auricular therapy, a practice related to acupuncture. Using a tiny electric current on specific points of the ear, we may eliminate cravings with the goal of allowing more effective healing.

I also recommend a specific dietary regime, including supplementation. Our goal is to help the body regain its chemical balance, restoring the brain's ability to accomplish the Brain Reward Cascade.

I believe this could enable patients to once again feel good about themselves without resorting to addictive behaviors and help break the cycle of addiction.

By breaking the cycle of addiction, patients can once again gain true health and wellness. As the philosopher Herophiles said in 300 B.C., "When health is absent, wisdom cannot reveal itself, art cannot become manifested, strength cannot be exerted, wealth is useless and reason is powerless."

This statement remains just as true 2,300 years later. And for addicts and others suffering from neurological problems, chiropractic care may open the door to newfound health and light the path to wellness.

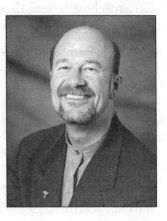

Dr. Brian Stearns, D.C., C.Ad.
AA Chiropractic, P.C.
3270 Market Street NE
Salem, Oregon 97301
(503) 364-9910

Dr. Brian R. Stearns, D.C., C.Ad. is a graduate of Northwestern College of Chiropractic, currently known as Northwestern Health Sciences University. He practices in Salem, Oregon and is licensed in Oregon, Washington State and registered in New South Wales, Australia. Dr. Stearns is active in The Oregon Doctors of Chiropractic (ODOC) having served as president twice. He is a Certified Addictionologist through the American College of Addictionology and Compulsive Disorders (ACACD).

Dr. Stearns is the proud father of three children and lives in Salem with his wife of twenty-one years. Before becoming a chiropractor, Dr. Stearns had driven dump trucks, fork lifts, bulldozers; built canoes, boats and pipe organs; dug ditches and been a performing musician. Through it all he realized that to perform optimally on any level, one must have all aspects (physical, mental-emotional, spiritual) of being intact. Body integration happens through the nervous system, which is what chiropractic and Dr. Stearns are all about. He has cared for individuals from two days old to ninety-nine years. He is currently in private practice, involved in research and has been published in several chiropractic journals and newspapers. Dr. Stearns has lectured for chiropractors and patients.

If you would like to schedule a private appointment with Dr. Stearns or arrange for him to speak to your corporation or group, he can be contacted in Salem, Oregon at (503) 364-9910.

PART FIVE

HEALTH: YOUR MOST PRECIOUS COMMODITY

Dr. Robert R. De Young II, D.C.
Dr. Maudie R. Louisiana, D.C.

Everyone defines success differently: a beautiful home, distinguished career, big paycheck, happy family, the adoration of others or whatever else we choose. It's possible to be a success in life, but a failure as a human being. Often we get so wrapped up in our careers achieving and attaining things that we ignore other areas of our lives.

Often we fail as people because we give up the most valuable asset we have — our health.

We give up responsibility and blindly turn over our health to someone else. We rely on hospitals, drug companies, insurance companies and even fast food chains to make choices for us.

Stop and think a minute. Is anything you have worth more than your or your family's health? Is there anything more valuable, more precious? Today I invite you to take a stand for yourself and your family. Take back your health!

Begin By Questioning Everything

First, examine the choices you make every day that affect your health. Spend more time researching health issues than you did buying your last car. Question the safety of the antibiotics, the Ritalin® and the vaccinations your children are getting. Question the prescriptions and over-the-counter medications you're on and find out how your doctor plans to get you off of them. Question any surgery or other radical procedure you may be considering.

According to a report published in the *Journal of the American Medical Association,* July 26, 2000, by Dr. Barbara Starfield, M.D., she states there is a total of 225,000 deaths per year caused unintentionally by treatments of medical doctors.

I feel there is a need, at times, for medicine or surgery, but these options should not become lifestyles. In my opinion, in the process of finding a quick fix, we are dying at an alarming rate.

Question the food you put in your body each day. Do you want a complexion, liver or heart made up of pesticide-laden, hormone-induced, antibiotic injected, partially hydrogenated cells? The cells that make up your organs and tissues undergo a constant, normal cycle of dying off and being replaced. The building blocks for new cells come from what we eat and drink every day. Coffee, soda, chips, sugar, fast food…many people ingest things they wouldn't even put in their pets' food dishes. They decide to put these substances in their own bodies. Stop and consider. You really are what you eat.

And most importantly, question where true health comes from. I believe each cell in the body has a tremendous force within it. This force was placed there by God and is called innate intelligence. Innate intelligence is your body's self-healing and self-regulating power.

For example, what happens if you cut yourself? You bleed. You may need a bandage or stitches; but eventually you clot and heal. Does the bandage or the stitches heal the cut? No, of course not. Your own body heals the cut.

And what if you fall and break your arm? Most likely you would need to get your arm set and a cast put on it. Does the cast heal your arm? Does the doctor who sets the bone heal your arm? No. Again, your body heals the fracture from within. The innate intelligence in your body heals your body. It happens no other way.

How Chiropractic Can Help

A woman came to our clinic after losing the use of her right shoulder for three years. She had undergone two complete rounds of physical therapy and two very painful cortisone shots with no relief. She admitted seeing a chiropractor was a last-ditch effort. She didn't know much about chiropractic care, but was willing to try. Recently she told us, "I'd say I have at least 85 percent use of my shoulder back! The bonus is not only has my shoulder healed itself through adjustments, but my menopausal side effects have greatly improved (night sweats, etc). My emotional welfare has also greatly improved. I am off anti-depressants for the first time in three years."

Every day we see people who have given up hope of ever having a normal life and feeling good again. Another patient of ours came in experiencing chronic neck pain, severe daily headaches and tingling in both arms and hands. These are the symptoms she was left with after two painful nerve root injections and a laminectomy (surgery where part of the vertebra is removed). She felt she had done everything she could and would have to learn to live in pain. After only two weeks of adjustments, the neck pain and tingling in her arms were reduced. In a few months, the headaches, neck pain and tingling were completely gone. To say she has a newfound zest for life is an understatement!

Another patient came in with an extensive history of knee pain. He had pain making it hard to go up or down stairs or lift anything. He was thinking he may need to have surgery. With chiropractic adjustments and some exercises the problem went away. In fact, after his knee was feeling better he said, "I had no excuse…I started walking on the treadmill, then running. I've lost 20 pounds. Also, I had been on medication for acid reflux for several years. That problem went away. I've been off the medication for eight months."

Yet another patient of ours wrote this: "After a month of coming to Your Life Chiropractic I've been able to throw away all my allergy medications. For the last three years I had been taking a combination of up to four allergy medications. Now I am medication-free and have so much more energy."

Some of our patients are most excited about other people's progress. When I asked one of our patients what has been the best thing she has experienced since her family has started care, she told me, "Witnessing my daughter have a normal life without migraine headaches. She missed a lot of school her senior year of high school. She started getting treatment and hasn't had a migraine since."

You should know these stories are TYPICAL of what happens in chiropractic offices every day. In each one of these cases the cause of their health problem was the same: subluxation.

Subluxation

Everything in the body depends on the communication flow of the nervous system, including innate intelligence. Anything that interferes with or diminishes the power of the nervous system could affect the power of innate intelligence. To protect such a vital part of the body, the brain and spinal cord are encased in solid bone, the skull and spine. Unfortunately, an unhealthy, injured or out-of-alignment spine can interfere with the nervous system. The most common cause of this is subluxation.

Subluxation is a tip or turn of the small bones of the spine, called the vertebrae. This misalignment puts pressure, traction or irritation on the nervous system.

According to studies done at the University of Colorado, subluxation can reduce nerve impulses by 50 percent. Another study found nearly 100 percent correlation between "minor curvatures" of the spine (subluxation) and diseases of the internal organs.

Capacity To Heal

Children are commonly known to heal quickly. You may have heard doctors say, "He's young. He should recover from this pretty well. Kids have a great capacity to heal."

Have you ever thought of where that capacity comes from, or what it is? We have already learned that this healing capacity of the body comes from our innate intelligence. But why do children have it in such supply?

Subluxations — the most common interference to the nervous system — are the cumulative result of chemical, physical and mental stresses around us. In my opinion, age typically results in more numerous and more advanced subluxations. Over time, subluxations go through phases of degeneration, causing the spine to deteriorate. But, the body maintains the potential power of innate intelligence.

So how do we sustain — or better yet — increase the power of innate intelligence? This is the question chiropractic sought to answer more than 100 years ago.

How do we increase the life force of the body? The answer may be by reducing or eliminating subluxation. It is the best kept health secret because most people have some degree of subluxation in their spines, yet few know it or what to do about it.

If subluxation is left undetected and uncorrected, it could diminish innate intelligence and possibly reduce health and ability to fight disease. Think of subluxation like this: Say your favorite radio station is 99.5 FM. If you tuned your radio to 99.3 FM., you may hear part of your favorite station, but most of what you hear would be static. This is what subluxation could do to the flow of the nervous system.

So what if subluxation was affecting the nerve to your hand, your thyroid gland, your lungs, your liver or maybe even your heart? If the nerve going to your hand was subluxated, it could cause numbness, weakness or possibly pain. If that nerve were going to your heart, it could cause some effect or strain on the heart.

Chiropractic works to eliminate subluxation from the spine and free the nervous system from interference. Specialized testing and X-ray examination can uncover areas of subluxation in the spine.

A chiropractic examination seeks to answer three basic questions: Do you have subluxation? If so, how long has it been there? And, can it be corrected?

If correction is possible, a chiropractic adjustment could reduce subluxation and restore normal flow to the nervous system. When normal flow is restored, innate intelligence could once again heal the body from within.

What are the big health concerns we have today? Cancer, heart disease and arthritis, to name a few. Despite decades of discovery, millions of dollars in research and numerous advances in treatments, these diseases have NO CURE. The only "cure" is to never get these diseases in the first place.

If your innate intelligence is working as it should, your body could be functioning at 100 percent. Your risk of developing these diseases could be much lower. Some of the healthiest people in the world get themselves and their families checked for subluxation with the goal of preventing disease from ever entering their lives.

So How About You?
The bottom line is your health and that of your family is the most precious commodity you have. Now is the time to take back your health and your life. Your health is not a one-time event. It is a process. Every day it's either increasing or decreasing, based on your actions — or lack thereof. If you would like to be healthier next year than you are right now, take action.

Don't put it off until New Year's Day or your next birthday. Don't even wait until Monday to change your life. Do it today! Question each and every health decision you make for yourself and your family. Clean up your diet. And for goodness sake, get a subluxation check-up!

> *"Or don't you know that your body is the temple of the*
> *Holy Spirit, who lives in you and was given to you by God?*
> *You do not belong to yourself, for God bought you with a*
> *high price. So you must honor God with your body."*
> – 1 Corinthians 6:19-20

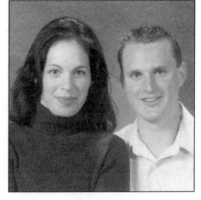

Dr. Maudie R. Louisiana, D.C.
Dr. Robert R. De Young II, D.C.
Your Life Chiropractic
103 Center Drive, Suite 200
Buffalo, Minnesota 55313
(763) 682-0611

Drs. De Young and Louisiana believe in natural health as the first choice, not the alternative. They are committed to creating healthy families through education, spinal correction and lifetime family wellnesscare. Both are founding members of Team Chiropractic Minnesota and lecture routinely on optimal health.

To schedule a private appointment with Dr. De Young or Dr. Louisiana or to arrange for either to speak to your corporation or group, call (763) 682-0611.

CHAPTER FIVE

ARTHRITIS
HEALTH SECRET

CHIROPRACTIC – A NATURAL APPROACH TO OSTEOARTHRITIS

❧

Dr. Dominique Dufour, D.C.

"I have nothing to lose!" These were Pierrette's words when she turned to chiropractic. Most patients with Pierrette's condition seek chiropractic as a last resort. She had been diagnosed with arthritis at the age of 40. Now 70, she had extensive hand deformity and increasing disabling joint stiffness accompanied by a general lack of mobility.

Pierrette was facing one of the most challenging situations of her life. She struggled with basic day-to-day needs such as eating, dressing and bathing. One of her greatest passions, playing the piano, was now a distant memory.

She was faced with the decision to either keep her house and freedom or move to a home which demanded less of her.

Pierrette was proactive with her health from the start. She had researched her condition and had read my articles in different publications. At first, people around her said she was wasting her time and money when she could be traveling and enjoying herself instead. But for Pierrette, traveling was not the solution to her condition. She chose chiropractic care in search of a better quality of life.

Ginette had extreme warnings her body was not functioning well. Her back had severe disc degeneration at cervical, lumbar and the mid-thoracic spine. At times the pain was so severe

Ginette could barely sit. Car rides were excruciating. She would lie on her back to minimize the jarring from road bumps.

Ginette followed my recommendations to the finest detail. This included: intensive chiropractic adjustments for several months to remove nerve irritation and promote cartilage regeneration, a detailed exercise program to rehabilitate and stabilize the spine and surrounding musculature, a positive attitude and appropriate nutrition.

Ginette and Pierrette now live lives their friends envy. These women faced their arthritic conditions and refused to believe nothing could be done. They encourage those around them not only to have their spinal health checked, but to bring their family members in for chiropractic care. They both say to me, "If only I had known before."

Chiropractic For Arthritis

Osteoarthritis is a common form of arthritis. The breakdown of cartilage could increase impact on associated bones. Stiffness, decreased mobility and joint aches can accompany osteoarthritis.

In Canada, one out of seven people are afflicted with arthritis. According to the University of Pittsburgh, 43 million Americans are affected by arthritis. It is estimated 70 percent to 90 percent of people older than age 75 are affected by osteoarthritis. Osteoarthritis can affect the whole body or specific joints.

This storm could be stopped and even prevented. I feel it is a matter of reducing the biomechanical imbalance by eliminating the stress that degrades the cartilage. Just like realigning a car with used tires, I believe reinstating a stable articulation will prevent further articular degeneration and the associated inflammatory crisis. One of the purposes of chiropractic is to realign joints. This could reduce pain and slow down the joint degeneration associated with arthritis. In addition to joints, arthritis affects the surrounding muscles, tendons and ligaments supporting the joints.

It is through the nervous system that the brain sends nerve impulses to communicate to the muscular system, the immune system and all the other systems of the body. Within this communication system, chiropractic identifies and corrects interferences, which are called subluxations. Removal of these interferences could allow the body to reinstate proper nerve flow.

Dr. David Felson, a rheumatologist from Boston University, comments on the arthritis disease process: "Everything is failing together. That includes bone damage, the responses to that, muscle weakness, inflammation of the lining of the joint and ligament disruption."

I believe for a treatment to be effective, all factors must be addressed. Chiropractic could be an excellent alternative to help deal with arthritis and maintain and reinstate harmonious, functional joints.

According to research published in *Topics in Clinical Chiropractic,* volume 3, number 2 entitled *Chiropractic Care Associated with Better Health in the Elderly,* 56.5 percent of patients who received chiropractic care on a prevention basis reported no arthritis compared to those not receiving chiropractic care who reported 34.3 percent not having arthritis.

This study also reported 87 percent of the adults receiving regular chiropractic care reported better overall health compared to 67.8 percent who did not receive regular chiropractic care. In addition, 52.2 percent of those receiving chiropractic care reported fewer chronic conditions than before they received chiropractic care. Of those not receiving chiropractic care, 37.1 percent reported fewer chronic health conditions. Regarding hospital stays, only 26.1 percent of those receiving chiropractic care reported stays in the hospital compared to 47.6 percent in the group not receiving chiropractic care.

I believe factors contributing to health are eating right, leading an active lifestyle, quality rest, a well-balanced psychological status and a functional nervous system. I feel chiropractic care is crucial in maintaining these factors in balance. Chiropractic care focuses on the body's innate healing ability to adapt to its environment.

A healthy, functioning spine and its associated joints could prevent premature degeneration by optimizing the flow of information to and from the brain. This helps ensure the body functions at its best, especially in arthritic patients.

Wellness-based care could be primary in preventing certain conditions like arthritis. Prevention could include identifying vertebral misalignment.

I do not measure health by the level of a person's physical activity. Often times, fit people are amazed by the degree of degeneration they see on their X-rays. "How can I have developed arthritis if I have been active my whole life?"

I believe exercise does not guarantee "healthy" joints. Waiting for pain could not be the best and most reliable indicator that something is wrong. I believe waiting for the condition to flare up is a mistake I see many people make.

Once the inflammatory state has set in, anti-inflammatory drugs are unfortunately the common route taken. According to a report published on November 10, 1997 by Stanford University School of Medicine, "Stomach bleeding is a well-known side effect of nonsteroidal anti-inflammatory drugs (NSAID), the most commonly used drugs in the world."

In the report, Dr. Gurkirpal Singh, a clinical assistant professor of medicine and senior research scholar at Stanford states, "More than 107,000 people are hospitalized every year in the United States for NSAID-related stomach bleeds and other complications, and 12 to 15 percent of those patients die from the bleeds." This means between 12,840 and 16,050 people die each year from NSAID use.

The body has the innate capacity to self-regulate, self-heal and self-regenerate. Some people turn to medication as a quick and easy "solution" for temporary relief of discomfort and pain.

Chiropractic views the body as a whole and not a sum of its individual parts. With this in mind, when I see a pain such as hip pain, I ask, "How could hip pain be localized and affect only the hip and not the entire body?"

To find the source of a problem, I view the body and nervous system as one entity.

You might find chiropractic practices that have surface EMG and thermography exams. Surface EMG can be used to detect electrical impulses sent from the central nervous system to the motor system (voluntary/muscular system). The infrared thermography reading gives temperature differential feedback of the autonomic nervous system and the related organs.

With orthopedic and neurological exams in conjunction with X-rays to view the spinal integrity and degree of degeneration, the chiropractor is able to determine the best protocol for the patient's well-being. Recommendations are established to relieve, correct, stabilize and prevent further degeneration and maintain a functioning and adapting nervous system.

Finding a quality of life means being able to appreciate the simple and pleasurable things in life. For Pierrette, it is being able to get dressed in the morning, play her piano and keep her independence without pain. For Ginette, it is being able to pick up and play with her grandkids and sit in the car rather than lay on her back for road trips.

Give yourself and your family the gift of life. To ensure an optimal functioning nervous system, get your spine checked regularly. I believe the power that made the body heals the body as long as there is no interference.

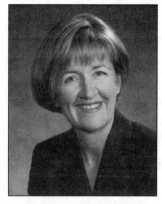

Dr. Dominique Dufour, D.C.
Clinique de l'arthrose
Clinique chiropratique
préventive et sportive
Phone (418) 687-5372
Fax (418) 687-5376
docteur.dufour@clinique-arthrose.com
www.clinique-arthrose.com

Dominique Dufour, D.C., founded Clinique de l'arthrose / Clinique chiropratique préventive et sportive in 1998. She obtained her Doctorate in Chiropractic from Logan College of Chiropractic in St. Louis, Missouri in 1980. Her mission for the past 25 years of practice has been to inform the community about health and wellness using a natural, chiropractic approach without the use of medication, surgery or medical intervention. She offers educational programs periodically to inform practice members and the rest of the population how to prevent, correct and stabilize arthritis.

Dr. Dufour has extended training certified in chiropractic occupational therapy (1986) and sports injuries (1986). She's a trained instructor in therapeutic touch (Touch for Health).

Dr. Dufour receives continued training in the latest scientific and technological developments in the field. In April and December 1994, Dr. Dufour and her staff received an honorary mention for their professionalism and service quality. Dr. Dufour was awarded the prestigious title of Chiropractor of the Year 2002 for the North American East Coast (United States and Canada).

She is a guest speaker at several organizations including the Association des arthritiques du Québec, the CLSC Haute-Ville, the Richelieu Club (Québec) and the YWCA. Dr. DuFour is a guest to conferences at Complexe G. In the past 5 years, she has appeared on a weekly television program, informing and educating the aging population about chiropractic. In addition, this past year, she had her own weekly chiropractic show focusing on the importance of quality of life and wellness.

She is a participant in the Programme des activités du 3e âge of the Université Laval and a geriatric pharmacology course presenting chiropractic as a solution to the excessive consumption of drugs.

CHAPTER SIX

SPORTS
HEALTH SECRET

The Wellness Secret: Chiropractic Care For The Working Athlete

Dr. Alfonso Di Carlo, D.C.

Many of us think of an athlete as someone young who participates in a vigorous, organized sport.

The truth is every one of us is a working athlete. Just meeting the incredible physical demands of everyday life requires peak conditioning from all bodies, young and old alike.

In my experience, there is a secret weapon used by countless professional athletes to give them the competitive edges they need. You might be surprised to learn it doesn't come in a bottle. It's called the nervous system.

According to the classic medical textbook, *Gray's Anatomy* (H. Gray, F.R.S., Chapter 1, Anatomy of the Human Body, 4), the nervous system's main function is …

"…to control and co-ordinate all the other organs and structures, and to relate the individual to his environment."

World's Best Kept Health Secret

In chiropractic, we believe health relates directly through the communication of the nervous system and that any interference in this system could affect the overall function of the body.

When interference occurs in the spine it is called vertebral subluxation. Regular chiropractic adjustments of subluxations, working in concert with good health habits, could free this interference. This may allow athletes' nervous systems to flow with less impediment, boosting performance and maximizing healing.

Many athletes depend on adjustments — from Arnold Schwarzenegger to Olympic Decathlon Gold medalist Dan O'Brien. These champions know that chiropractic's proper application goes well beyond the usual stereotype of simply relieving back pain.

Deepak Chopra, M.D. coined the phrases, "Health is our natural state" and "All disease results from an interruption to the flow of intelligence." With proper adjustments, adults and children alike could experience a surge of renewed vigor by tapping into their innate intelligence.

Why do top athletes get regular chiropractic care? Dr. Anthony Lauro and Dr. Brian Mouch produced a comparison study entitled *Chiropractic Effects on Athletic Ability* with 50 athletes participating. They were divided into two groups. One group received chiropractic care. The other served as the control group and did not receive chiropractic care. Eleven tests were used to measure athletic abilities such as agility, balance, kinesthetic perception, power and reaction time.

After six weeks, the control group without chiropractic care showed minor improvement in eight of the 11 tests. The group of athletes who received chiropractic care improved significantly in all 11 tests. In the hand reaction test, the control group exhibited less than one percent response. The group of athletes receiving chiropractic care exhibited more than an 18 percent response after six weeks. After 12 weeks, the chiropractic group exhibited more than 30 percent improvement. Maybe that's why the world heavyweight boxing champion Evander Holyfield stated in *Today's Chiropractic* Magazine, "I have to have my adjustment before I get in the ring."

From the moment we're born and for decades afterwards, our bodies could be subjected to untold physical, chemical, and emotional stressors. Unfortunately, these stressors might even cause subluxations within children's young spines.

The birth process itself may be the first cause of interference within the nervous system. According to Dr. G. Gutmann, in his research titled, *Blocked Atlantal Nerve Syndrome in Babies and Infants,* (Gutmann, Manuelle Medizin, 25:5-10, 1987) from his and other medical studies, Gutmann concluded that approximately 80 percent of all children are not in autonomic balance and that many have atlas blockage or subluxation.

This study stressed the importance of having infants' necks (specifically the atlas) examined shortly after birth, especially if the birth was a difficult one. Dr. Gutmann states over 1,000 children were treated successfully, almost without exception, for a variety of ailments by spinal adjustments at the atlas.

Dr. Gutmann quoted another study that examined 1,250 babies five days after birth. Of this group, 211 suffered from vomiting, hyperactivity and sleeplessness. Upon examination, 95 percent of these children had upper cervical atlas strain. Release of this strain by chiropractic adjustment "frequently resulted in immediate quieting, cessation of crying, muscular relaxation" and the children typically fell asleep.

And Dr. Abraham Towbin, in his work *Latent Spinal Cord and Brain Stem Injury in Newborn Infant,* (Develop, Med., Child Neurol.,1969,11:54-78), "Forceful longitudinal traction during delivery, particularly when combined with flexion and torsion of the vertebral axis, is thought to be the most important cause of neonatal spinal injury. It is evident that a close relationship exists between the traction stress applied and the occurrence of spinal lesions. When excessive traction is applied to the fetal spinal column, fracture, dislocation and cord transection occurs. It is unlikely that these lesions, under these circumstances, are attributable to pathologic processes other than the applied traction stress. Traumatic damage to the spinal structures is not an all-or-none condition; the occurrence of neonatal spinal fracture with cord transection following excessive traction is a fact from which it follows that lesions of less severity also occur as a result of forceful traction."

A young person's body is undergoing tremendous changes during the crucial period of childhood and adolescence. In order to have a strong immune system, you may want to consider the nervous system needs to be in prime working order at all times.

According to Dr. David Felton, M.D., Ph.D., "Nerve fibers go into virtually every organ of the immune system and form direct contacts with the immune system cells…" (B. Moyers, *Healing and the Mind,* New York: Doubleday, 1993).

Furthermore, Dr. Seth Sharpless of the University of Colorado reminds us that all it takes is a miniscule amount of pressure on a nerve, about 10 mm Hg, which is equal to a feather falling on your hand, to reduce the function of the nerve by up to 50 percent.

Olympic Aspirations

As an exercise and sports science specialist, I know that, along with the alignment of the spine, focusing on the alignment of extremities could help kids achieve proper balance. It could also reduce stress on young joints and aid in helping achieve optimum physiology of movement in their athletic fields of endeavor.

To illustrate, I'd like to introduce two of my young patient athletes: Bryce, age 12, and his brother Dale "DJ" Winterhoff, age 14. Starting their racing careers in downtown Chicago, this dynamic duo trained for, and won, a combined total of nine gold, nine silver and eight bronze medals in IronKids competitions across the country.

At early ages, they mimicked their father who was training for triathlons. Now in their adolescence, the Winterhoff boys keep a constant eye on someday achieving Olympic Gold. They have been interviewed on television networks such as ESPN, Nickelodeon GAS and PBS. Their role models include their good friend and U.S. Olympian Hunter Kemper, who also came up through IronKids and is currently ranked 8th in the world.

In spite of their superior physical condition and their amazing achievements, these brothers regularly schedule chiropractic adjustments to realign subluxated vertebrae with the goal of restoring proper nerve function to the body.

According to the boys, they no longer worry about one of their legs working harder in a distance run than the other one. Nor do they find themselves drifting into the lane lines during a swimming competition. With each correction, the boys feel as if their nervous systems are operating at peak performance.

In fact, Bryce, who was an 11-year-old national triathlon champion, asks for an adjustment before every race. He wants to know, from the starting line, that no stone has been left unturned in the pursuit of winning.

The boys no longer get sick when working out intensely all year nor do they miss practice sessions. The Olympic Team has a saying, "It's not every four years, it's every day." The Winterhoff boys take those words to heart.

They are now training for the 2012 Olympics. Their winning team includes their parents, coaches and me as their chiropractor. These athletes agree wholeheartedly with Dan O'Brien who said, "If it wasn't for chiropractic, I wouldn't have won the gold medal." (December, 1999; *The Chiropractic Journal*)

I believe every working athlete should be checked for subluxations before, during and after training sessions to keep fit and injury-free with the goal of extending the longevity of his or her athletic career.

Planning A Healthy Future

Chiropractic wellnesscare is effective. I feel parents must insist on making this issue a community and family affair. Mothers and fathers could give their budding Tiger Woods and Lance Armstrongs real head starts by having children participate in chiropractic adjustment plans. For the child athlete, I believe it is a good move for parents to ask school sports programs and neighborhood athletic organizations to have a team chiropractor who is providing care with the goal of lessening the likelihood of injuries.

The importance of staying healthy is paramount. According to the U.S. Consumer Product Safety Commission, 2,804,118 children were seen for sports related injuries in 2002.

Here's how you can get started. First, don't wait until your child gets sick or injured. Schedule a chiropractic appointment for your whole family today. Your son or daughter's body is growing right now and likely pushing itself to its limits through this growth. Then add the further demands sports can bring. There is a clear need for chiropractic. In fact, many extracurricular activities such as playing a musical instrument, studying or just surviving the pressures of young adulthood could possibly cause subluxations that need to be addressed.

After the initial family consultation, I recommend you keep regular appointments through every stage of your family's growth and development, even if you all lead a symptom-free life.

The cost of healthcare nationwide might be greatly reduced if only more people understood about the healing strength of their own bodies, a strength that could be rediscovered at your chiropractor's office.

The wellness secret is out! According to a study published in *Journal of American Medical Association,* 1998;280:1569-1575 entitled *Trends in Alternative Medicine Use in the United States, 1990-1997* conducted by Dr. David Eisenberg, M.D. and associates, " . . . a 47.3 percent increase in total visits to alternative medicine practitioners, from 427 million in 1990 to 629 million in 1997, thereby exceeding total visits to all U.S. primary care physicians."

The study went on to say, "The visits to practitioners of alternative therapy in 1997 exceeded the projected number of visits to all primary care physicians in the United States by estimate 243 million."

According to world-renowned economist Paul Zane Pilzer, we are entering the "Wellness Revolution."

In 1975, Dr. Ronald Pero, Ph.D., chief of cancer prevention research at New York's Preventative Medicine Institute and professor of medicine in Enviromental Health at New York University, studied 107 people who had received long-term chiropractic care. According to the report, the chiropractic patients in his study had no obvious reasons for increased susceptibility or resistance to disease. The report states, "the chiropractic patients also had 200% greater immune-competence than people who had not received chiropractic, and 400% greater immune-competence than people with cancer or other serious diseases."

During the study, the competence of the immune systems did not decline with age. The health of the immune systems in the study remained uniform for the entire group regardless of age.

Pero concluded, "chiropractic may optimize whatever genetic abilities you have" to fight serious disease. He continued, "I am very excited to see that without chemical intervention…this particular group of patients under chiropractic care did show a very improved response."

Dr. Pero, who has published over 160 papers in medical peer review journals, firmly believes chiropractic care was the key factor in this study.

Maybe that's why so many top athletes get regular chiropractic care. Professional athletes understand **the world's best kept health secret!** But don't just take my word for it. Listen to what five time Cycling Champion Lance Armstrong says in the book *Every Second Counts*, "The team wasn't just the riders. It was the mechanics, masseurs, chefs, soigneurs and doctors. **But the most important man on the team may have been our chiropractor.**"

Now could be the time for parents to recognize new methods available for children and take action! Whether you are out there after Olympic Gold or shuttling around a carload of future Olympians, chiropractic offers a safe, all-natural way to unleash your inner champion for the entire family.

"The fundamental reason why people struggle to achieve optimal health is because they search on the outside. The result is people continue to spend money in search of the latest product, but never learn that health and wellness comes from WITHIN!"

– Dr. Alfonso Di Carlo

Dr. Alfonso Di Carlo,
D.C. with IronKids®
champions Dale "DJ"
and Bryce Winterhoff

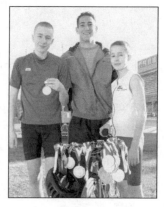

Dr. Alfonso Di Carlo, D.C.
C.A.F.E. of Life Chiropractic
2059 Route 309
Allentown, Pennsylvania 18104
(610) 366-1336
doctordicarlo@hotmail.com

Dr. Alfonso Di Carlo, a Penn State University graduate with a degree in Exercise Physiology and Sports Science, focuses on athletes and lifetime family care. He specializes in corrective care of the nervous system and alignment of the extremities. Dr. Di Carlo has a passion for working with children and helping them experience active, healthy lives by promoting regular chiropractic check-ups. Since 2001, Dr. Di Carlo has hosted the worldwide Kids Day America/International event in Allentown, PA.

Explore the fact your health comes from within! Go ahead...call Dr. Di Carlo now at (610) 366-1336 or visit www.wellnesssecret.com and learn more about how the wellness secret can help increase your health and vitality!

PART TWO

Chiropractic For The Competitive Edge

Dr. Patrick Baker, D.C.
Dr. Paul Baker, D.C.

From professional athletes to weekend warriors, we believe the spine must be in 100 percent alignment to achieve peak athletic performance. Simply put, 100 percent alignment could equal 100 percent function.

A subluxation, which is a misaligned spinal vertebra, could cause a decrease in speed, range of motion, flexibility or endurance and possibly increase the risk of injury during athletic endeavors.

At our practice, my brother and I treat a number of professional athletes from all sports for a variety of injuries including, but not limited to shoulder and knee injuries, back strains and pulled hamstrings.

We developed and trademarked a new approach to treating muscle injuries called Muscle Injury Release Technique (MIRT™). The goal of MIRT™ is to strip away old scar tissue, relieve pain and facilitate healing.

MIRT™ works toward eliminating scar tissue formed between muscle fibers (also called fibrotic adhesions). This is important because not only could scar tissue contain more pain fibers than healthy tissue, but also could inhibit the injured muscle from healing properly.

The growth of scar tissue follows a natural physiological process with devastating effects. When we injure a muscle, scarred muscle tissue moves along the muscle belly and adheres to the tendons at the origin and insertion points of the muscle. This is actually a protective device to enable the movement of a larger area of muscle groups while restricting or immobilizing smaller groups.

How can a person tell if he has scar tissue? The most common way is to move the joint and the affected muscle. Signs of scar tissue may include:

- Trouble moving the joint and injured muscle through different ranges of motion,
- Decreased muscle strength,
- Premature fatiguing of the injured muscle.

Releasing scar tissue through MIRT™ is crucial to helping the body regain its maximum potential. While a fairly new procedure, MIRT™ has shown a high success rate in treating thousands of muscle injuries during the past few years. MIRT™ involves no surgical procedures, no artificial equipment and no medications. It is a technique of skill involving the doctor's hands and/or elbows working in an intense, rhythmic and aggressive motion to strip away old scar tissue and generate long-term pain relief.

Football Player Finds Relief

In 2001, Corey Dillon, a Cincinnati Bengal and two-time Pro Bowl running back from the National Football League, entered our clinic complaining of chronic pain in his right hamstring. It was the result of an injury suffered in 1994. Since the injury, this professional athlete underwent traditional massage therapy, physical therapy, electrical stimulation, injections and the use of pain relievers – none of which brought him the relief he sought.

An examination of his hamstring revealed a build-up of scar tissue the size of a tennis ball. We implemented MIRT™ for an intense 15 minutes and the knot began to disappear.

This course of treatment took multiple visits. We now perform pre and post game structural corrections (adjustments) and MIRT™ for this professional athlete and a number of other professional athletes.

MIRT™ can be uncomfortable at first, but some patients could feel immediate and substantial pain relief after the first treatment. Subsequent treatments are less uncomfortable, and after two to three MIRT™ sessions, patients could experience strong differences in flexibility, joint mobility and pain relief.

Not Just For Football Players

Whether the injury is a hurt shoulder, strained pectoral muscle, lower back spasm or any other muscle injury, MIRT™ could strip away the build-up of scar tissue so that the muscle has a chance to heal correctly. When an injury occurs or when a muscle tightens up through a repetitive motion (like throwing, running or weightlifting), the body automatically attempts to self-heal by sending extra blood to the area, producing swelling.

Swelling cuts off the oxygen supply to the muscles and connective tissues producing a condition called hypoxia. As a result, flexibility of the muscles and joints is severely limited. Oftentimes, patients know they are in pain, but do not realize they have built-up scar tissue that could be relieved by MIRT™.

We believe the reason we see so many professional athletes is because they may be becoming increasingly disenchanted with the typical allopathic medical treatments they are receiving. My brother and I find as these athletes receive chiropractic, they begin to realize they could achieve wellness – a wellness approach traditional allopathic medical treatments may not provide for them.

However, professional athletes are not the only people who could suffer sports-related injuries. In fact, we feel it is the weekend warrior who could be more prone to injury than the well-conditioned professional athlete. The most common injury we see among weekend warriors is to the lower back. This could be because of the weakened spinal musculature in the lower back. Lower back muscles may become weak or de-conditioned over time, making a person prone to misaligned vertebrae or subluxation. This could result in a painful pinched nerve.

The principal sign would be a pain in the lower back. A more severe sign or symptom could be waves of pain down one or both legs known as sciatica. Sciatic pain is often felt in the lower back and along the back of the thigh and could involve one or both legs.

Four Step Process

Chiropractic treatments (adjustments) over a period of time can be essential for strengthening the lower lumbar spinal musculature. We can align the vertebrae, but weak lower back musculature won't hold the spine's alignment. To maintain the alignment, we stress the need to rehabilitate and strengthen lower back muscles. We work with our patients to help them strengthen their lower back muscles through a complete rehabilitation program.

This is part of our four-step wellness program: chiropractic care, exercise, massage therapy and nutrition. This four-pronged approach is our wellness program. We believe it is important to realize you cannot get to wellness unless these four methodologies are practiced routinely.

One of our patients entered our clinic nearly 100 pounds overweight with severe lower back pain and leg pain. By adhering to our chiropractic wellness protocol, we alleviated the patient's back pain, and the patient lost 94 pounds by following our exercise program and nutrition plan. This case demonstrates the life-improving changes one could achieve by following a dedicated plan that leads to wellness without the use of dangerous drugs or surgery.

We admit some of our patients find our program very challenging. But as they say, nothing good ever comes easy. We realize it is a major challenge for someone to go through a paradigm shift from sicknesscare to wellnesscare. We believe wellnesscare is feeling good and maintaining 100 percent function without having to take medications.

To help patients understand the benefits of shifting from sickness to wellnesscare, each and every patient entering our clinic goes through a four-day education process on chiropractic care, traditional medical care, nutrition and exercise.

The goal of our education protocol is to help the patient understand the differences between allopathic care (sicknesscare) and chiropractic wellnesscare and to convert them from a sickness symptomatic care mindset to a wellnesscare mindset.

This is not always an easy task. Americans have been bombarded since they were little kids with television and radio marketing messages advocating pills to cure illnesses. Everyday the airwaves are filled with commercials touting a pain-relieving pill for everything from arthritis to migraines. Our education process explains and teaches that wellness comes from within the body, not from outside. Once patients understand and adopt this philosophical change, they often become long-term chiropractic wellness patients.

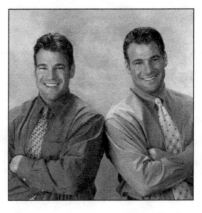

Dr. Patrick Baker, D.C.
Dr. Paul Baker, D.C.
Baker Family Chiropractic
4781 Red Bank Road
Cincinnati, Ohio
Phone (513) 561-2273
Fax (513) 561-3571
Dokbonz@aol.com
www.bakerfamilychiropractic.com

Drs. Patrick and Paul Baker are Ohio natives and have been practicing chiropractic in the Cincinnati area since 1993. The doctors bring over 20 years of chiropractic experience and soft tissue healing techniques to their thousands of patients. Graduates of Palmer College of Chiropractic in Davenport, Iowa, they bring eight years of college and over 500 hours of continuing education in physical rehabilitation, sports injuries, nutrition, athletic training and permanent spinal impairment ratings.

The doctors are nationally recognized for founding and developing a revolutionary soft tissue healing technique known as **MIRT**™ — Muscle Injury Release Technique. Many professional athletes from all over the country consult the Bakers' for the doctors' soft tissue healing expertise.

Both doctors are active members of the American Chiropractic Association, International Chiropractic Association and the Ohio State Chiropractic Association.

In their spare time, the doctors lecture nationally on chiropractic, nutrition, athletic training and sports injury rehabilitation. Both doctors are former award winning bodybuilders and bodybuilding judges for the National Physique Committee.

CHAPTER SEVEN

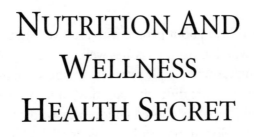

NUTRITION AND WELLNESS HEALTH SECRET

PART ONE

WELL-ADJUSTED LIVING

❧

Dr. James D. Eckert, D.C., L.C.P. (Hon)

We often hear about people who are "well-adjusted." These are people who handle life's issues well.

Amazingly, some people receive this label even though their lives have been more difficult than most of us realize. There are people who started as abused children or who grew up in the slums, yet developed into positive role models. They refused to be victims or give up. These people realized it is not so much *what* happens to them. It is how they respond. Their successes are determined by their choices, not by the environment or "the hand they were dealt."

Such stories give us hope and teach us what is possible when we are true to the best *in* us, rather than focusing on outside circumstances. When we are true to ourselves, we can reach our potential, regardless of circumstances or what others think. Isn't that what we want for ourselves and our families?

These people demonstrate a life principle known as "Above-Down, Inside-Out" (ADIO). This is the realization that everything good in our lives comes from God "Above" and "Down" to us.

If we are open, it will then come from "Inside" us to "Out," becoming a reality. People who live this way do not allow outside influences to determine who they are inside their skin or what they will do. Living this way allows us to stay true to God and ourselves. It will ultimately lead to living the lives we were meant to live.

Conversely, many people mistakenly believe and live their lives with an "Outside-In, Down-Above" approach. They spend their whole lives searching for health, wealth and happiness. Often, they never find it. Why? I believe it is because they are looking in the wrong places, *outside* of themselves. They try to use *outside* influences to change what they don't like *inside* themselves and their lives, rather than change themselves. They want to do it their own way regardless of the laws of life. Like gravity, these laws of life exist and govern independent of anyone's opinion or belief. It is not our choice whether they exist or what they are, but our choice is whether we work with or against them.

Examples of these "outside-in" behaviors are:

- Pursuing health through outside means. An example could be initially turning to medications, procedures, lotions and potions without proactively creating preventative wellness *inside*. A person in this situation may wait to notice his or her health until it begins to decline *outside*. This is very dangerous because many diseases start without any outward symptoms at all.
- Wealth by chance or some stroke of luck.
- Happiness attained through possessions and other people.

All of these approaches rely on things outside of us. This takes away our power and says we cannot accomplish success by ourselves. We cannot heal ourselves, become financially independent or decide to be happy without certain people or possessions.

I believe the "outside-in" approach never works. Why? I have never known anyone to be truly happy or healthy when approaching life and health from the outside-in. Because of my experience and my understanding of some of the laws of life, I believe happiness and health only come *from within*.

ADIO From The Beginning

I believe life began for you at the moment of your conception. This miracle called life has an innate or inborn intelligence which caused a few cells to multiply into trillions. This innate intelligence naturally knew what you needed when you needed it in order to become you. Everything progresses as it should unless something interferes with this natural process.

Within a short period of time from conception, as the number of cells grew, your innate intelligence needed a system to send and receive messages. The purpose of this system was and is to control and coordinate all functions and parts of the body. It is called the nervous system. Being so valuable and delicate, the nervous system's primary parts, the brain and spinal cord, are the only organs encased in bone.

Innate intelligence carries messages from the brain above and down through the spinal cord. It flows from inside your body out to all parts.

What would happen if this intelligence flowing by way of vital messages through the nervous systems could not reach the intended body organ in the right amounts at the right time? What if interferences blocked messages on how to function sent from your brain to your heart, lungs, liver, kidneys or stomach? Could this affect your organs and your ability to function to the highest potential?

Functioning Potential Examined

Life and health are dependent on our ability to adapt to the stresses of life. People make efforts to decrease stress, which can be difficult. In my opinion, it is more important how we *respond* and *adapt* to stressors. Our ability to respond and adapt is dependent upon the uninterrupted flow of the nervous system. It stands to reason when nerve flow is interrupted our ability to function and adapt could be reduced. Do you think this could make us more susceptible to illness and injury?

How Does This Happen?

Subluxations are misalignments of spinal bones which interfere with the nerves as they exit the spine. Since all body functions are controlled and coordinated through the nerve system, without proper nerve flow, body function would be compromised.

How do subluxations or "disruptions in the flow" occur?

The nerve system gets overloaded with physical, chemical or emotional stressors and could cause spinal bones to subluxate or misalign. A "short circuit" in the nerve system or "a disruption of the flow of intelligence" often results.

Subluxations of the spine are the most common disruptions to the flow of innate intelligence. Can you truly be healthy if you don't keep your spine free from subluxations for life?

When do many people get their first subluxation? We now know many people will get their first subluxation at birth. According to Abraham Towbin, M.D. from Harvard Medical School, "During the final extraction of the fetus (baby), mechanical stress imposed by obstetrical manipulation – even the application of standard orthodox procedures — may prove intolerable to the fetus."

Furthermore, Dr. Towbin states, "Spinal cord and brainstem injuries *occur often* during the process of birth, but *frequently escape diagnosis*...there may be lasting neurological defects."

Therefore, it's no surprise chiropractic care should begin at birth on a preventative basis.

The Four Essentials Of Life

Current research tells us it is not so much our genes that determine our health, but the expression of those genes. This could be largely dependent on our lifestyle choices and how we address the "four essentials" of life and health.

Most people are aware of the first three: food, water, oxygen. Fewer are aware nerve function is one of the four essentials.

To figure out the order of importance, ask yourself how long you could live when each is taken away. Without food, you could live a few weeks. Without water, a few days. Without oxygen, a few minutes. But without nerve function, you could die immediately.

You need to have all four essentials or you wouldn't be alive. It is not a question of whether you have them. It is a question of quality.

I want to see people have true health through high quality essentials. If essentials are not available or cared for, it is no accident when problems develop.

For example, if we ate junk food rather than healthy food every day, would it affect our health? Clearly it affects our health and can likely shorten our life as well.

Poor quality oxygen or smoking will affect our health and might cut our lives short.

Many health problems I see in my patients are due to lifestyle choices. Heart disease from poor diets. Lung cancer from smoking. Tooth or spinal decay from neglect.

Just because you eat right and exercise doesn't mean your nervous system is free of subluxations. And just because you keep your spine and nerve system free from subluxations doesn't mean you can eat junk food and become a couch potato.

Conditions resulting from bad habits usually take years to develop and the symptoms often only appear after extensive damage has already occurred.

You have the opportunity to change the way you take care of your health. I recommend a change from believing you are well just because you feel fine to knowing health is not about how you are feeling, but how you are functioning.

The longer subluxations are left, the more spinal decay could be created. Decay results from years of neglect and/or abuse. Pain and symptoms often only appear in more advanced stages of the decay process. Should you wait for pain to show up before you consider your spinal health? What would you do if your spine wears out? Remember, your spine is irreplaceable!

To minimize the effects of subluxations and avoid spinal decay, consider including chiropractic care in your lifestyle.

As a Doctor of Chiropractic, my goal is for your body to perform the way it is supposed to — at its best! No matter age or level of health, everyone should be checked for subluxations to make sure their nerves are functioning properly.

Since subluxations are misalignments, what do you think is the only way to correct them? Of course, the answer is to realign them through chiropractic adjustments. For this reason chiropractic is not an "alternative," but a unique solution to a common problem — subluxation. Chiropractic adjustments could help you to adapt, heal and perform at your best. Are you "well-adjusted?"

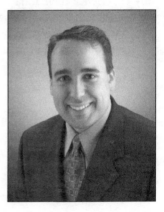

Dr. James D. Eckert, D.C., L.C.P. (Hon)
Innate Chiropractic
210 Western Avenue
South Portland, Maine 04106
(207) 775-7468
drjim@innatedoctors.com
www.innatedoctors.com

At 27, Dr. Jim Eckert received his Doctorate of Chiropractic degree from Palmer College of Chiropractic where he graduated with honors. By the relatively young age of 33, Dr. Jim Eckert became a noted chiropractor, educator, speaker and writer. He has established a state-of-the-art, award winning practice being recognized among chiropractic offices across the eastern United States for his "Faithful Devotion and Exceptional Service to his Patients, Community and the Chiropractic Profession." His office is one of the first in the country to implement and utilize the Creating Wellness System™, a three-dimensional approach to health and wellness incorporating not only the physical and biochemical aspects of wellness, but the psychological component as well.

Dr. Jim Eckert has received a postgraduate certificate for Paraspinal Electromyographic and Thermographic scanning. In addition, he has also furthered his education by receiving his Legion of Chiropractic Philosophers degree, an advanced, post-graduate, honorary degree in the philosophy of chiropractic giving him an in depth understanding of the natural laws that govern health and healing.

He is passionate about sharing the chiropractic message with humanity. So he is actively involved in advancing chiropractic and its principles locally, across the country and around the globe by actively participating in multiple chiropractic organizations. These include the Maine Chiropractic Association, the Chiropractic Leadership Alliance, the Federation of Straight Chiropractors and Organizations, the World Chiropractic Alliance and the International Chiropractors Association (ICA). He is a founding member of the ICA Council on Chiropractic Philosophy and is committed to helping people understand chiropractic principles so they may not only improve their health, but also their lives.

His life mission is to help everyone realize, continually express and fully experience their innate potential in health and life by correcting subluxations and enlightening minds.

To schedule a private appointment with Dr. Eckert or to book him to speak for your corporation or group, call (207) 775-7468.

PART TWO

WELLNESS CARE:
UK AND AROUND THE WORLD

❧

Dr. Christian H.E. Farthing, BAppSc (ClinSc); BCSc
Chiropractor (Australia) • Spinal Specialist (United Kingdom)

Do you really think headaches are due to an aspirin shortage in the body? Do you really feel ear infections are due to a lack of antibiotics in the body? Do you even believe hay fever is a shortage of antihistamines in the body?

In my opinion, this type of thinking is so ridiculous it borders on the humorous.

But when was the last time you reached for an anti-inflammatory or muscle relaxant for back pain or some other malady? Did the tablet have the word "back" written on it? How did that tablet know where to go in your body to relieve your pain?

I see the problem with all of this is our belief system. When we were younger we may have suffered with a headache and so were given medication. The headache went away. This may have happened a few times, over a number of years to the point where every time we had a headache, we reached for a tablet of some kind. Why? Because it relieved the pain. But did it address the *cause* of the pain?

Does It Really Work?

The belief that a pill is the answer to every pain, symptom or other body signal creates a behavior. A behavior so common, you may not even question it.

Massive advertising campaigns by drug and pharmaceutical companies may lead some to believe pills might be harmless. Our behavior may then become acceptable within the community. So accepted that it creates a social environment with thousands to millions of people turning to pills and tablets for relief.

The irony of all this is, with all the technology, research and money invested into our healthcare system, it does not appear to me we are any healthier.

So much time and money have been invested in understanding sickness and disease. The "real solution", I believe, should come from understanding what we need to do to create health and wellness.

To change our social environment and behavior, I feel we must first change our beliefs understanding health and healing come from within. Sickness and disease manifest themselves on the inside of the body. Therefore to regain health, wouldn't a focus on healing from inside of the body make sense?

Wellness is a further manifestation of moving towards optimal health from within the body. We need to realize health comes from a body functioning the best way possible on the inside.

Health From Within

Have you ever wondered what healthcare and wellness really mean? Does the word "medicine" sound like healthcare to you? To me, it seems often when people go to the doctor they are given some form of pill, potion or shot.

This has been described as the 'law of addition by subtraction'. To me, this means when you are sick, you are prescribed something — in other words, something is added to the body.

If this doesn't work, you may undergo testing to reach a diagnosis. Then you could be given another form of medication. If your symptoms do not improve, your medication might change or you might be given something else. You may even be given different medications to offset the side effects of other pills you have been taking.

If your condition does not begin to improve and your body signals persist, you may be asked to have a surgery to remove or "subtract" a dysfunctional part of your body.

This philosophy works on adding foreign substances to the body with the hope of alleviating your symptoms. It may or may not correct the cause. If all else fails, the option may be to remove a part of your body.

How have we come to believe this is okay? Do we really have any spare body parts to remove?

Looking At The System

According to research conducted by University College London and reported by *The Sunday Times,* medical error is the third most frequent cause of death in Britain after cancer and heart disease, killing up to 40,000 people a year – about four times more than those who die from all other types of accidents.

Provisional research figures on hospital mistakes show that roughly 280,000 people suffer from non-fatal drug-prescribing errors, overdoses and infections. These people spend an average of six extra days recovering in hospitals, at an annual cost of 730 million pounds in England alone.

Is the system working? Is it time for our beliefs, behaviors and social environment to change? I believe the answer is "yes." I see a health revolution occurring.

I believe more people each year are turning to health providers who look for causes, rather than treat symptoms.

Have you ever wondered what would happen to a healthy person if you gave them medication? Would they possibly become ill?

So why, then, is the answer to give medication (that is foreign to the body) to a sick person and expect to them to get healthy? Are there any other choices? The solution to having other choices is to have other beliefs.

I believe health and healing occur from inside the body, rather than from the outside. This principle has been around for many years. It is coming to the forefront of health and wellness. This principle is so powerful it could transform the whole idea about how to get well and stay well.

I see healthcare and wellnesscare as being about keeping you healthy — not solely warding off sickness. Wellness is part of the healthcare revolution — a revelation!

So how do you find wellness? What steps can you take to function better? How can you live with greater health and vitality? How can you restore your health and move towards wellness?

Healthy Nervous System

Because the brain and central nervous system control all body functions. To operate at optimal levels, I recommend you ensure your body has 100 percent nerve flow — free of interference.

It is when there is obstruction to this life force and life giving nerve flow that we could be predisposed to sickness and suffering. Nerve interference could reduce immune function, decrease your energy and productivity and cause muscle weakness, pain, headaches, numbness and so much more.

Nerve interference in the body is caused commonly by a condition known as vertebral subluxation. This is a misalignment in the spine that puts pressure on the nerves, resulting in nerve interference. Subluxations can go undetected for years without symptoms. They could begin to compromise your health and wellness.

To have a better chance at life, as I see it, you should make sure your spine is in good alignment. The spinal cord and nerves act as your lifeline and transmit messages to and from the brain. That is why I believe a healthy spine, free of subluxations, means better communication within your body and a healthier nervous system. This could mean optimal function and better health inside your body.

So, to make a difference in your health and the health of your family, children, friends and loved ones in Australia, the United States or Canada speak to a Doctor of Chiropractic. In the UK, speak to a Chiropractor or Spinal Specialist who are specifically trained in the detection and correction of vertebral subluxation.

The wellness revolution is here. Every year around the world an increasing number of people are becoming aware of the amazing benefits of chiropractic care and spinal care. People are discovering the benefits of natural health and wellness.

The New England Journal of Medicine published a survey by Dr. David Eisenberg, M.D., of Boston's Beth Israel Hospital, which reported one-third of American adults are going outside of American mainstream medicine and using alternative healthcare methods. People understand they have health and wellnesscare options.

Unfortunately, in my opinion, the UK appears to be behind in the area of wellness. Chiropractic was founded in 1895, but chiropractic care in the UK is still in its youth. Worldwide, chiropractic is the largest, drug-free healing profession and the third largest healthcare profession.

In the UK, a movement is occurring to answer the many questions people have been asking. I made a decision to continue the high standards provided by the leading chiropractors around the world. As a Doctor of Chiropractic in Australia and a Spinal Specialist in the UK, I share the best kept health secret with my patients and community on a daily basis.

This gift was given to me when I was only six months old and I had my first subluxation check-up. And so I give it to you...the revelation of wellness and the best kept health secret...to use, enjoy and share with all those around you.

May your health continue to improve and flourish as you move toward greater wellness in your life. God Bless.

Dr. Christian H.E. Farthing, BAppSc (ClinSc); BCSc
Chiropractor (Australia)
Spinal Specialist (United Kingdom)
Ideal Spine Centre
30 Whitstable Road
Blean, Nr Canterbury
Kent, United Kingdom CT2 9EB
+44 (0)1227-789-977
www.optimalspine.co.uk
wellness@optimalspine.co.uk

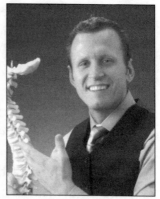

Dr. Farthing has been a chiropractic patient since he was six months old. His mother, Valerie, a trained nurse, understood many years ago that the birth process can be traumatic to the spine of newborns, and how important a healthy spine and nervous system are for growth, development and optimal health. Therefore, she took her son for his first evaluation. Since then, Dr. Farthing has grown to understand wellnesscare first hand, having regular spinal check-ups throughout his life. It is now his mission to share this "health secret" and way of life with his patients and community.

Dr. Farthing now practices as a Spinal Specialist in Blean, near Canterbury in Kent in the United Kingdom. His speciality in the detection and correction of the most common form of nerve stress, vertebral subluxation, has made him well-known around the world. His commitment to providing a service to his patients and community has allowed him to create one of the busiest spinal and subluxation-based practices in the UK.

He has a vision and commitment to creating a healthier community, educating and adjusting as many families as possible toward optimal health and wellness through modern natural spinal care.

Dr. Farthing wants the public to receive the highest standard of healthcare that is among the fastest growing, natural forms of healthcare around the world. He has spent the last 10 years studying and practicing the principles of optimal performance health and healing and spinal correction. This, and the deteriorating health in the community, inspired him to create a health practice providing superior facilities with affordable, modern natural healthcare for families.

The Ideal Spine Centre was designed and built to provide solutions to the many unanswered health problems so many people experience every day in their lives. It is a unique health practice that is not only a healing environment, but also an educational institution to empower people to make better health choices and understand what true health and wellness really is.

To schedule a private appointment with Dr. Farthing or to arrange for him to speak to your corporation or group, call +44 (0)1227-789-977.

BEST KEPT
HEALTH SECRET

❧

Dr. Jonathan Lemler, D.C.

This secret goes against our society's tendency to always try to *add* things to a problem in order to "fix" it. Headache? Add aspirin. Depression? Add anti-depression medication. Swelling? Add anti-inflammatory medication.

This health secret identifies the most important thing to *subtract* or eliminate from a health problem.

What Is That?

Interference within the master controller of the body, the nervous system. We call this interference a "subluxation", which at its root meaning translates as less (sub) light (lux). It is caused directly by spinal misalignments or dysfunctions where the vertebral bones are out of place or not moving properly and could result in nerve irritation.

In a manner of speaking, you might say we do not have enough light in our bodies when we have subluxations. Light is energy. The brain communicates through the nervous system to all the cells, tissues, organs, glands and muscles of the body.

Basic physiology tells us the energy along the nerve is electrical and chemical in nature. When there is a disruption of this flow of energy, like a vertebra creating irritation to a nerve, there is something partially or completely (as in quadriplegia) blocking this "energy" or light. This results in a shadow being cast, so to speak. We are "dimmer." And we also feel like a "shadow of ourselves" as a result!

Common Causes

What causes vertebra to subluxate and irritate the nerves, dimming the lights?

Traditional healthcare does not take subluxation into consideration when dealing with health problems. They never bother to look at *all* the causes of subluxations. They may address a few issues like diet, but they rarely do it comprehensively. Therefore, you could be left with incomplete healthcare. Or, at best, short term symptomatic improvement, but a continued breakdown of the body.

First you can categorize the types of causes, as many have done, into four main stress categories: physical, chemical, environmental and energetic (mental, emotional and spiritual).

Within the physical stress category you would find accidents, falls, injuries, the birth process, postural habits (such as how and what you sit on), work activities and exercise habits, etc.

Chemical stressors include what you eat, the water you drink, the air you breathe, the supplements or medications you take and mercury in dental amalgam and vaccinations.

Environmental stressors include cold, damp weather, electromagnetic pollution (such as high tension power lines or pulsed radar), too much UV radiation and ozone depletion and obvious toxic chemicals from internal combustion engines, manufacturing waste and pesticides, etc.

How do chemical stresses cause subluxations? They chemically irritate the body's tissues which could set up a chain reaction in the nervous system creating feedback tension in the muscles. This may pull on the spinal vertebrae creating a spinal malfunction or, more accurately, further misalignment and malfunction.

Subluxations can just build up. After the initial subluxation event, like a car accident, birth trauma or even some type of poisoning, all subsequent events could create greater nerve irritation and interference.

Now, if this interference involves the nerve going to the liver, for example, that could create less liver function. The liver eliminates poisons and toxins from the body.

What could happen if the liver is not fully functioning? If you eat something contaminated with a heavy metal or you are exposed to a pesticide, a compromised liver is not as able to remove toxins from the body. Toxins may accumulate, creating damage. This could lead to a greater degree of nerve irritation and subluxation!

You may have no clue how your liver is functioning right now. If you have some kind of advanced liver disease, you may see your skin turning yellow or your blood tests may show a high level of certain liver enzymes. Otherwise, it may be a challenge for you to determine the health of your liver.

Chiropractors could identify the potential for irritation to tissues by evaluating you for subluxations. If you have a subluxation at a certain level of the spine, you may have nerve irritation at that level. This could result in less light, energy or nerve impulses to the tissues.

You may or may not have a disease yet. Disease is in the realm of medicine. Chiropractic deals with dis-ease, a lack of ease and light. You may or may not have an outward symptom, but you still may have an underlying subluxation.

Another stressor is energetic or mental, emotional and spiritual stress. Do you know someone who worries so much he or she becomes sick with an ulcer or headache? That is a simple example of this type of stress. This process takes a thought (worry) and creates a physiological reaction related to the nature of the thought and the condition of the individual such as a weak digestive or muscular system. The same stress could create different effects depending on the individual's make-up and pre-disposition.

Why is this considered an energetic cause of subluxation? Because the mental, emotional and spiritual realms are not matter, or physical substance, but are energy. Remember $E=mc^2$? Things are either physical or chemical matter or they are energy. Mental energy is manifested in our thoughts. Our emotions are our feelings and could create significant good or bad physiological reactions.

Without getting too esoteric, I believe your spiritual state is at the foundation of all of this. This connection or disconnection to a higher Source could result in a greater or lesser sense of purpose. This could affect the meaning of life and the will to persevere.

As said by D.D. Palmer, the founder of chiropractic, the purpose of chiropractic was to "unite man the physical with man the spiritual." Once we are united in this way, life is more joyful and fulfilling. We all benefit from a better and deeper connection to our spiritual source.

What can we do about these stressors?

12 Secret Keys To Outrageous Health And Prosperous Living

The first secret key is to realign and reconnect the structure. I believe a chiropractor is by far the most qualified to do this. Without this, the other 11 Keys are not nearly as effective as they could be.

Secret Key 1:   Realigning and reconnecting the structure.

Secret Key 2:   Detoxification and drainage — removing the "crud" to open space inside for the good stuff.

Secret Key 3:   Individualized assessment of eating, diet and lifestyle choices.

Secret Key 4:   Replenishing lost or low nutrient levels.

Secret Key 5:   Balancing organ, gland and tissue systems.

Secret Key 6:   Rebuilding and supporting the immune system.

Secret Key 7:   Evaluating and correcting electromagnetic influences.

Secret Key 8:   Addressing other environmental issues such as water, air, toxins, etc.

Secret Key 9:   Establishing exercise, movement and fitness activities.

Secret Key 10:   Releasing and healing mental and emotional pains and stresses.

Secret Key 11:   Enhancing personal potential and abilities, attracting prosperity and abundance.

Secret Key 12:   Reconnecting spiritually.

Where do you start? Prioritize according to your individual needs. I feel Secret Keys One and 12 are absolute musts. Then you can address numbers two through 11 in the order you deem best for you.

Chiropractors correct subluxation. We use many methods to do this such as our hands or special adjusting instruments. The goal is a less stressed nervous system. This could give the body a chance to use more of its internal energy for repair and rejuvenation, not to mention a more efficient metabolism.

I've discovered in order to maintain a spinal adjustment or correction, people must have properly nourished and strong connective tissue, which holds your body together.

Protein, the main element of collagen, is the essential ingredient in connective tissue. Unfortunately, our society is overfed and undernourished. Our protein sources are typically unhealthy or overcooked, which breaks down the essential amino acid proteins which are the building blocks for collagen.

What are your options for receiving sufficient protein to help form healthy connective tissue and maintain chiropractic adjustments?

I have found a good source is undenatured whey protein. I make sure it has not been heated past a certain temperature so the amino acids are not broken down.

As you become more connected physically and spiritually, you attain a higher level of knowingness. As you apply this greater sense of knowingness to your decisions to take action on a daily basis, you attain a higher level of wisdom. The good actions you take will result in the life benefits you seek.

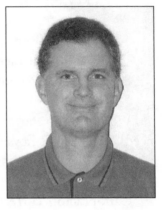

Dr. Jonathan D. Lemler, D.C.
Healing Arts Center
1259 West Gonzales Road
Oxnard, California 93036
(805) 485-1802
drjlemlerdc@earthlink.net
www.HelpCare4U.com

Dr. Jonathan Lemler, D.C., (aka The Health Answer Man), is a sought after expert, speaker and media guest. He received his Bachelor degree in Biology from UCLA and graduated Summa cum Laude from the Los Angeles College of Chiropractic with his Doctorate of Chiropractic.

He is in his 24th year as Founder and Director of the Healing Arts Center of Ventura County, California, where the latest health and wellness technologies are combined with traditional touch therapies to deliver true health and well-being. The Health Answer Man welcomes your health questions at DrjLemlerDC@earthlink.net . If you would like to schedule a private appointment with Dr. Lemler or arrange for him to speak to your corporation or group, call (805) 485-1802.

PART FOUR

GOOD HEALTH BEGINS WITH YOU

Dr. Brent Baldasare, D.C.

There is something you value above all else. You rarely think about it until you lose it.

It's something you pray for when your new baby is born. You toast to it when you gather with friends and family. It's your greatest asset or your biggest downfall.

What Is It? Your Health.

Being healthy is something we all want, but only a small percentage of us take the proper action to achieve. The typical person does so little to ensure health and so much to damage it.

One of my favorite comedians, Steve Martin, was introducing a handsome young Academy Award winner to the stage and said, "I would do anything to look like that...except eat right and exercise."

How true that is for most of us. We want to look better. We want to feel better. We want to be healthier. But we lack the motivation or knowledge to reach our goals.

Some people may wish good health and vitality could come in a pill, a drink or a chocolate-covered bar. A quick fix. Achieving good health is not a quick fix. It's a lifestyle of making good choices about your food, your healthcare team and which bad habits to release.

Getting Started

Whatever level of health or personal development you want to achieve, it starts with how you perceive yourself accomplishing it. I had a college football coach who had us mentally rehearse tackling the opposing quarterback. Our coach was mentally preparing us by visualizing our success.

The night before we played Georgetown University, I remember dreaming of getting to the quarterback over and over. During the game, I had four quarterback sacks, which was a season high. Success happened long before the actual game. Mentally, I had already accomplished my goal.

At some point in your life, you may begin to realize your level of health is up to you. If you can visualize yourself in a smaller size, you could get there. I personally believe if you visualize your body overcoming a disease, you could do it. You'll have people who tell you otherwise. Obstacles are what we see when we take our eyes off goals.

If you are healthy, you likely have a lifestyle of good habits. If your health is fleeting or you're constantly sick, I hope today you make a choice to improve your condition for good.

If becoming healthy or improving your body is a high priority, there are specific steps to ensure you have the best chance of success. The first action step is having a plan. Consulting with a wellness chiropractor is a good place to start.

Improving the lives of others is my life's passion. I want every person I meet to understand what it means to be truly healthy. I want people to increase the quality of their lives without sacrificing simple enjoyments. I promote healthy habits, but I am not a fanatic.

My definition of a perfect state of health is when all areas of a person's life are at optimum levels. You have to take care of yourself physically, mentally and emotionally. When I talk to patients in my office about being healthy, it's important we agree on the definition of health. A lot of patients say they think their health is fine because they feel good.

They say things like, "I don't have pain anywhere" or "My cholesterol and blood pressure are fine."

Below is the exact medical definition from *Dorland's Medical Dictionary:*

Health (**health**) (helth): a state of optimal physical, mental, and social well-being, and not merely the absence of disease and infirmity. **Holistic Health:** a system of preventive medicine that takes into account the whole individual, his own responsibility for his well-being and the total influences—social, psychological, environmental— that affect health, including nutrition, exercise, and mental relaxation.

Healthy Profile

The healthiest people in the world have common characteristics. First, they make time for themselves.

I remember reading Lee Iacocca's book. During his presidency at Ford Motor Co., Mr. Iacocca would not hire executives unless they took vacation time. Mr. Iacocca understood healthy people can be among the most highly productive.

Healthy people think positively. They exercise regularly and handle stress well. Healthy people eat regular meals and wholesome foods. They drink lots of fresh water daily. They have healthy nervous systems, which can help them function at higher levels.

Research attributes a significant amount of diseases to stress. Stress is created by how we perceive or handle the environment around us. There are three major stress factors: physical, chemical and emotional. Together they form the "Health Triangle":

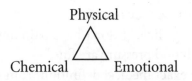

Physical

Chemical   Emotional

Each corner in the triangle represents a major stress factor. If any of these areas are out of balance, it could result in declining health. For example, emotional stress could lead to digestive problems, which could create physical stress. In turn, this could cause chemical dependency to medication.

If the root cause of the stress is not found and removed, a dangerous pattern of ongoing self or prescribed medication might possibly elevate this situation. I believe a whole body or holistic approach must be taken.

Overcoming Stress

We all have stressors in our lives such as family situations and financial matters. How we handle stress determines if our health improves or declines.

After I have evaluated the state of my patients' health, there are specific habits I want all my patients to include in their daily routines, if physically appropriate for their conditions.

- Begin a resistance training exercise program three days a week for thirty to forty-five minutes. The benefits of this one habit for people of all ages are enormous.
- Develop healthy eating habits. Foods that don't perish on the counter don't digest well in the body.
- Reward yourself for doing well. Being a fanatic on any plan leads to early burnout and loss of interest.
- Increase your fresh water intake. Water purifies the body and rids toxins.
- Get your rest. You need to let your body recharge to keep you strong and healthy.
- Reconnect with your spiritual side. Either through prayer,

meditation or reaffirmation of faith. Longevity studies at the University of Colorado have shown, in general, those who have a deeply rooted faith and attend religious services one or more times each week live about seven years longer than those who never attend. The study was found to be the same for all faiths.

- Enjoy yourself. Don't take yourself too seriously.
- Commit to the plan prescribed by your chiropractor or other wellness doctor. Don't just dabble. Keep to your purpose and give your plan for health all you can. You need to be responsible for your own well-being. It's up to you to stick to the plan.

Remember, achieving health is a process. Finding a wellness chiropractor is a start. And keeping fun and happiness in your life is the secret to your success.

"My vision is to create a safe, wholesome environment for drug-free healing. The world is full of overmedicated and sick people who need our help. True health comes from within and we tap into that potential with every adjustment."

— Dr. Brent Baldasare

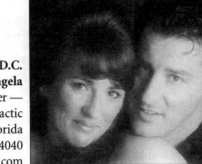

Dr. Brent Baldasare, D.C.
and wife Angela
Affinity Healthcare Center —
Family Chiropractic
Orlando, Florida
407-381-4040
www.affinityhealthcarecenter.com

Born in Linwood, New Jersey, Dr. Baldasare is licensed by the Florida Board of Chiropractic.

He received his B.S. degree from Ursinus College in Philadelphia, Pennsylvania and his Doctorate of Chiropractic from Life University in Atlanta, Georgia. His internship was completed in Atlanta, Georgia specializing in pediatric chiropractic and family wellness. His externship was completed in Orlando, Florida specializing in personal and sports injuries.

Dr. Baldasare is a member of the Florida Chiropractic Association, the American Chiropractic Association, the International Chiropractors Association, the World Chiropractic Alliance and the Florida Chiropractic Society.

Dr. Brent Baldasare first experienced chiropractic after a paralyzing college football injury. He lives in Orlando, Florida with his wife and three children. He is the Clinic Director and Owner of Affinity Healthcare Center. To contact the author, Dr. Baldasare can be reached at 407-381-4040 or visit www.affinityhealthcarecenter.com .

PART FIVE

BODY BALANCE – A KEY TO WELLNESS

Dr. Gary F. Loranger, D.C.

A fine-tuned body, like a fine-tuned machine, functions better, breaks down less often and lasts longer.

I believe we should strive for balance in our lives — in everything we are and in everything we do.

We need to balance:

- Sleep with the amount of time we're awake,
- Work with time we spend playing and relaxing,
- Calories we consume with calories we expend through exercise,
- Time we spend alone with time we spend with friends,
- Time we spend with friends with time we spend with family,
- Satisfaction of carnal needs with satisfaction of spiritual needs,
- Receiving with giving,
- What we earn and what we spend.

Imbalance in our physical, emotional or spiritual being could create instability and stress in our lives. Physically, we need to maintain balance in our musculoskeletal (muscles and bones) system. We need to maintain normal balance and alignment of our joints and muscles, which comprise our body's posture. A normal, balanced posture is necessary for normal function of our muscles and joints.

I believe abnormal posture and dysfunction of muscles and joints could cause irritations to the body's nervous system. Could these irritants contribute to a breakdown in wellness? The irritations I refer to are otherwise called subluxations, which could be corrected with chiropractic care. By balancing the body's spine and postural musculoskeletal system with chiropractic adjustments, irritation could be removed from the nervous system. This might aid the body to function and heal as I feel it was designed.

Master System

The nervous system has been referred to as the "Master System" of our bodies because it controls and coordinates the function of all other systems, keeping them organized and functioning properly.

I see health as a condition or state of the body in which every organ, tissue, cell and gland is capable of performing the function for which it was designed to do. All systems of the body depend upon a normal functioning nervous system and an uninterrupted flow of nerve impulses from the brain. I believe it is necessary for complete communication to exist between the brain and the rest of the body in order to maintain optimum wellness. This communication is accomplished through *nerve transmission* from the brain to all tissues of the body by way of the spinal cord and spinal nerves. To maintain wellness it is vital that no interference exists with the transmission of nerve impulses coming from and going to the brain.

The spinal cord runs down from the base of the skull to the lower back. The spinal cord transmits nerve impulses from the brain to all of the organs and tissues of the body. Thirty-one pairs of spinal nerves branch off from the spinal cord, with one pair between each of the vertebrae of the spinal column. These spinal nerves carry the nerve impulses from the brain to all of the organs and tissues of the body and then from organs and tissues back to the brain. The spinal cord and spinal nerves are the conductors of nerve impulse transmissions. These impulses, generated by the central nervous system (the brain and spinal cord), are the energies that keep us healthy and alive and in tune with ourselves and our environment. The ability of this energy to flow freely throughout our bodies without interference from subluxations is the goal of chiropractic care.

I feel traditional medical care is directed more toward treating diseases or symptoms of diseases. In my practice, chiropractic care is directed at restoring proper joint and muscle function, spinal alignment and normal body posture and mechanics. Removing interferences or subluxations of the nervous system is the objective of my care of patients. A chiropractic analysis is made not to "name a disease." Rather, I desire to detect the presence of imbalance and dysfunction in the body causing nervous system irritation.

Chiropractic For Wellness

Many people mistakenly think chiropractic care is only a treatment for back pain. Although spinal adjustment of subluxations can be one of the most effective treatments for back and neck pain, chiropractic care offers much more. My central interest has always been the relationship between subluxations and the nervous system. Chiropractic adjustments not only correct local spinal problems that may cause back pain, but could also influence other body functions and dis-ease states through nerve reflex mechanisms. I believe chiropractic adjustments can have an impact on a variety of nerve pathways between the spine and the organs that regulate general health.

I feel keeping the body in balance and free of subluxations so its nervous system can coordinate proper function is the reason many people make periodic visits to their chiropractors.

Chiropractic concerns itself with the proper balance, alignment and function of the musculoskeletal system – the body's posture. In my practice, particular attention is directed toward the spine and the cranium since they house and protect the central nervous system – the brain and spinal cord. I feel the structure and function of your entire body is associated with a normally balanced and functioning spinal column because of its intimate relationship with the nervous and musculoskeletal system.

Could people be suffering due to subluxations in their spinal column? Abnormal spinal alignment and function could be the result of a lack in proper spinal care. I believe regular chiropractic visits could help counteract the accumulation of stresses and strains on our bodies from activities of daily living.

Any machine that gets a great deal of use, and often abuse, will go out of adjustment from time-to-time and could require a "tune-up." Our body is no exception. The gradual accumulation of the seemingly minor stresses and strains our bodies are subjected to on a daily basis, if not cleared, could eventually overcome the body's ability to adapt and may result in pain and other dysfunction syndromes. I use chiropractic adjustments to help "clear" the accumulated stresses, which could enable the nervous system to coordinate health without interference.

Do I Have To See A Chiropractor Forever?

No, you definitely do not have to go forever. Once a person's initial problem is fixed, the doctor may release him or her from care. How long it takes to correct and stabilize a spine-related problem depends on many factors. In my practice, treatment is directed toward attaining postural balance, restoring normal spinal mechanics, stabilizing joint and muscle function, and relieving nervous system irritation. Some cases could be managed in as little as a few days. Others in a few weeks. Some may require a few months or more of care. Each individual case is unique.

As a Doctor of Chiropractic, I don't prescribe "lifetime" care to anyone for the correction of any musculoskeletal disorder. You may have been led to believe you have to go to a chiropractor forever. Whether a person chooses to continue visiting his or her chiropractor for preventive-maintenance care after the initial problem is corrected is entirely up to each person.

What Is Preventive-Maintenance Care?
I feel "healthcare" is doing things necessary to take care of oneself in an attempt to prevent pain, sickness and disease. I believe true healthcare is a conscious, self-directed effort and plan carried out to enhance and maintain optimal body function.

I feel people sometimes take for granted everything will work properly in their bodies without doing anything to enhance and maintain their health. We may have been conditioned into believing when something goes wrong and we become sick or feel pain, all we have to do is get a prescription and all will be well again. I believe going to a doctor only when something hurts or when we become sick is not healthcare – it's sickcare. I also feel this could be a very dangerous approach to caring for ourselves. Could utilizing such an approach increase your risk of developing future health problems? This may be why people don't feel as well as they could.

There Is A Better Way
In my practice, the reason many people visit my office regularly is not because they "have to," but because they choose to. I believe they understand the value of taking care of themselves when feeling healthy in order to help prevent unhealthy conditions from afflicting them. Also, they seem to understand maintaining the body in a healthy state makes more sense than waiting until they have a health problem before seeking care.

I believe people who visit their chiropractor regularly understand and appreciate the important relationship their spinal postural/musculoskeletal system has to the nervous system and the vital role that relationship can have in restoring, enhancing and maintaining their health.

The Chiropractic Choice

In my office, lifetime preventive-maintenance care, or wellnesscare, is intended to maintain the body in its optimal functional state of well-being and to help prevent the development of abnormal spinal conditions and spinal nerve stress disorders. Lack of proper spine and posture care could be the reason spine-related disorders are high in our society.

I believe a healthy immune system allows the body to heal itself and to maintain good health as long as there are no interferences or subluxations blocking its ability to do so.

I believe drug therapy could aid the body in recovery when administered at the appropriate time and for the appropriate reason when someone whose own natural disease fighting mechanisms have become overwhelmed. I feel drug therapy should be reserved as a last line of defense.

In my office, the use of chiropractic adjustments may allow a person's body a chance to heal on its own. I also believe by removing interferences or subluxations using chiropractic adjustments instead of drug therapy, the body's disease fighting mechanisms could strengthen and allow the body to heal naturally. Untreated subluxations could adversely affect general health and wellness of the body's nerve reflexes. Chiropractic adjustments could remove the interferences in the nervous system and may improve the overall function of the body. Regular chiropractic adjustments could keep the body in balance — "fine-tuned" — free of subluxations, postural distortion and consequent nervous system irritation. Chiropractic adjustments may influence a variety of nerve pathways that regulate general health.

I feel chiropractic wellnesscare is one of the best and truest healthcare practices available today. By keeping the structural/

mechanical integrity of the body in balance with regular chiropractic care, people are able to enjoy the benefits of a balanced body, free of subluxations, taking their health to higher levels and maintaining it.

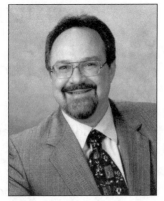

Dr. Gary F. Loranger, D.C.
Loranger Chiropractic Body
Balance Center
1811 King Road
Trenton, Michigan 48183
(734)675-7090
drgary@forbodybalance.com
www.forbodybalance.com

To schedule a private appointment with Dr. Loranger or to arrange for Dr. Loranger to speak to your corporation or group, call (734) 675-7090.

PART SIX

OPTIMIZE YOUR HEALTH

Dr. Glenn Gabai, D.C.

As an individual, what is the single most important thing to you?

A number of people might answer their families are most important. They might be able to name several instances where they have placed their families' needs before their own.

Other people might answer that their jobs are the cornerstones of financial support for their families. Others might say happiness is the most important. Yet others might say life itself is most important.

All of these could be correct answers. However, underlying them is a deeper and more vital most "important thing." What is it?

Health. Think about it. Everything you do seems dependent upon having your health in order to accomplish it.

Since health is so important, where do you think health comes from? Many would say it comes from eating well, proper supplements or getting enough water. Others might say health is about attitude, exercise and the ability to deal with stress. Others feel "taking proper care of the body" will bring health.

Does health come solely from external choices and sources? Or could health also come from within?

Basis Of Chiropractic Science

I feel life and health are based on the inborn innate intelligence of the body. How do our bodies function? Could it be an intelligent power controlling body cell and nervous system functions? Could an unlimited supply of energy, an intelligent powerhouse, reside in the living brain?

I believe innate intelligence flourishes within us from the moment of conception to what is perceived as death. I see it as the guiding force as nutrients assimilate and cells divide. Could it be as you are reading this right now that innate intelligence is directing your metabolism, creating new cells and controlling your heartbeat?

Life sustaining energy starts in the brain and flows through the central nervous system throughout the body. Could it be the difference between a healthy, fully functional human and a diseased human is the quantity and quality of life energy reaching the cells?

Chiropractic Body

What is the most important part of the body? Could it be the heart and its functions? Or the brain or lungs? Every part is the most important part of your body. Here's why. When the heart, lungs, spine and brain are perfectly healthy but the body is unable to eliminate wastes, how long before health is out of balance?

With all parts of your body having significance, could your life and health depend on every organ doing its job 100 percent properly? And what exactly is 100 percent function of any one organ? Can we really understand every single function of any one organ of the body?

The job of the brain and nerve system is to control and coordinate all the other parts of the body. The word for this is homeostasis — the maintaining of the internal environment. This involves feedback from the entire body, the monitoring of thousands of events every second and the regulating of each and every tissue with the goal of 100 percent normal function.

What else does the brain do? The brain thinks. The higher level function of our thinking makes us unique as a species.

However, the most important function of the brain is the most elusive to understand.

What is the difference between a living body and a corpse? They both have the same body parts. What the live body has, that is missing from the dead body, is life energy or vital force. The Eastern philosophies call it chi. It is what animates the living body and is the only difference between the living body and the corpse.

The Inside-Out Job. Exactly Who Is The Boss?

What does your body do? The job of the body is to do what your brain directs. It is a vehicle for your purpose. Who decides your purpose? You do.

If you wake up in the morning with the flu, will you be able to live your purpose to the best of your abilities?

Many times people feel they function normally with the body out of balance, but symptoms could affect our abilities even if we think otherwise. Could you do better for yourself than simply learning to live with symptoms? Is it normal to have to live your life with symptoms rather than health?

The job of the brain is controlling and coordinating the body while thinking and producing life energy. What connects the brain with the body? The nervous system.

Physiologists call the nervous system the master control system of the body.

How does it work? If you step on a tack, how does the brain know it? The brain sends the controlling coordinating messages to the body. The organs then send messages back to the brain for the feedback mechanism to be complete.

As you are reading this you are breathing, digesting your food and your heart is beating without you even thinking about it. Though you may not know what this master control system is all about, you are dependent upon it every moment of your life.

It is my experience that human mental impulse is unlimited,

exhaustless and dependable from conception to death. Ease or coordination is a manifestation of harmonious action of all the body parts, each fulfilling its purpose. With information flowing back and forth between brain and body via nerves, proper or normal body function could be a reality. What is this? HEALTH.

BRAIN ➠ NERVES ➠ BODY ➠ 100 PERCENT FUNCTION ➠ EASE = HEALTH

Vertebral subluxation is a misalignment of spinal bones. This could create irritating pressure on the spinal cord, nerve roots or tissues surrounding the nerves. Such irritation might affect the energy flowing through the nerves.

I define life as the presence of vital energy flow to and from the brain. I see this vital nerve impulse as electrochemical energy. It could be affected by physical or chemical irritation caused by spinal bones or discs out of normal alignment.

BRAIN ➠ NERVES ➠ BODY ➠ malfunction ➠ disEASE = SYMPTOMS

Spinal vertebrae protect the soft spinal cord and nerve fibers just as the skull protects the brain. A vertebra out of normal position could alter nerve function and ability to carry messages between the brain and body.

Vertebral subluxation is similar to having a pebble in your shoe. The pebble is a physical thing causing pressure and irritation on a nerve. It may even become painful.

What would you have to do? Remove the pebble, take off the shoe and give the body time to heal.

Subluxations could be similar. The nervous system, when free of interference, could provide for proper physical and mental function and efficient adaptation to the environment.

I describe vertebral interference as having five components:
- Abnormal motion or position of the spine,
- Abnormal nerve function,
- Abnormal muscle function,
- Abnormal tissue function and
- Resultant degenerative changes.

If normal function creates the state of ease or comfort, then altered function could be termed dis-ease or discomfort.

What Can You Do To Optimize Health?

As you quietly read these lines, a whirl of activity is taking place in your body without your conscious effort. Every second new tissue cells are created in the body's ceaseless program of self-renewal. I believe the same intelligence that created a live animal from a single fertilized ovum maintains that matter in existence. Could this master controller have superimposed its intent, purpose and design into every mental impulse and nerve force flow?

Subluxations

There are many causes of subluxation. The general categories are:

- Physical (falls, car accidents, posture),
- Mental (stress, tension, worry, aggravation),
- Chemical (poor nutrition, smoking, alcohol, drugs).

Chiropractors remove subluxations safely and systematically. Chiropractic spinal adjustments involve aligning the spine and removing potential interference to health expression.

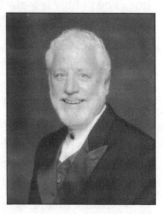

Dr. Glenn Gabai, D.C.
Pennington Family Chiropractic
2554 Pennington Road
Pennington, New Jersey 08534
(609) 737-3737
e.gabai@att.net
www.familychiropractic.com

To schedule a private appointment with Dr. Gabai or to have him speak for your corporation or group call (609) 737-3737.

PART SEVEN

THE MIND-BODY CONNECTION

Dr. Elliott J. Mantell, D.C.

"Each patient carries his own doctor inside of him. We are at our best when we give the doctor who resides within each patient a chance to work." – Albert Schweitzer, M.D.

What is the mind-body connection and how does it relate to our health?

David was 59 years old when he first came to my office. He had been suffering from depression, allergies and knee and back pain for almost 20 years. Although he had been on anti-depressant medication for the past two years, he still felt depressed more frequently than he could tolerate. David was equally concerned about the drug's side effects and his lowered state of energy.

David reported that within the first month of starting chiropractic care, he stopped taking his medication. One month later, he reported he felt better than he had in years — with or without medication. He began an active exercise program and within a few months had the motivation to climb Mt. Hood and Mt. Adams. No small achievement at any age.

Whether we're conscious of it or not, we innately recognize the remarkable mind-body connection and interaction. We cannot deny the power of the autonomic nervous system, which keeps us breathing, digesting and living life while we go on about our daily activities.

We all know someone who has suffered from "tension headaches," stomach ulcers and heartburn that flare up at times of stress. These are examples of the body automatically responding to mental and emotional states in distinctively physical ways.

We can become especially vulnerable to accidents, injuries, colds, flu or fatigue during difficult times. We can all sympathize with the mental and emotional stresses created by a prolonged illness or chronic pain.

The mind-body connection is undeniably present and active in our lives. But are there ways to actually use this connection to our advantage? Can our understanding of this connection help us enjoy vibrant good health, faster physical recovery, decreased pain, a higher state of consciousness and an improved quality of life? After over 20 years of experience caring for people in wide-ranging states of health, I know it can!

Yet few people consider the mind-body connection when facing specific health challenges. What's more, many patients tend to panic at the onset of a symptom and go to invasive extremes. When they feel a knot forming in a muscle or a headache coming on, they often attempt to use force or drugs to stifle it. But heavy-duty treatments may not be the answer and may actually ignore the root of the problem.

Drugs and forceful techniques may only repress the symptoms our bodies have generated to alert us of disorders within. In order to truly honor the mind-body connection, perhaps we should seek to make use of the symptom, whatever it is, as an entryway into deeper healing.

For many patients, the lightest chiropractic care touches may present the mind-body connection. That's why I facilitate my patients' healings through a specialized form of chiropractic care called Network Spinal Analysis (NSA). NSA is a synergistic blending of the most successful chiropractic techniques developed over the past 109 years. It is supported by the latest discoveries in quantum physics, neurology and mind-body medicine. With the gentlest of contacts, the use of this healing art could enable patients' bodies to naturally heal from within by reinforcing the innate mind-body connection.

The brain is the master coordinator of the body, communicating to each organ and cell through the spinal cord. In fact, the spinal cord is not separate from, but is a continuation of the brain. Fluid known as cerebral spinal fluid transmits chemical information to and from the brain and affects the tension or "tuning" of the whole nervous system. It also flows all the way down to our lower spine (sacrum). Any disturbance to this bodily system could affect our health.

So when stress or injuries result in distortion patterns or subluxation to the spine, the mind-body connection could also be affected.

Since the brain and spinal cord control the entire body, any disturbance to our communication system could prevent us from being our best. Subluxations, which can be caused by physical trauma, accidents, injuries or emotional stress, could block the flow of nerve impulses from the brain to the body. The results could be devastating to our bodies physically, as well as affect us mentally and emotionally.

Take my patient, Vania. At 28 years old, she was injured in an automobile accident and was experiencing neck, jaw and shoulder pain as a result. After only one month of care, she felt less physical tension and more relaxation in her muscles. Interestingly, once her physical symptoms began to clear, Vania said, "Physically, I felt less tension and more relaxation in my muscles as well as an increase in breath from my spine into my brain. Mentally, I feel more alert, focused and present. Emotionally, I feel more able to deal with stress and have a better overall sense of well-being."

Our work rests on a firm foundation of excellent chiropractic care. The original tenets of chiropractic held that mechanical disturbances in the spine and nervous system could affect the optimum functioning of our vitalistic innate intelligence, thus interfering with overall health and well-being.

The Network Spinal Analysis approach addresses disturbances in the nervous system and assists the body in developing
self-regulating processes to remedy tension contributing to the
individual's overall wellness. Many people compare NSA care to
an upgrade of computer software or an invisible boost to nervous system efficiency to better handle an increasingly fast-paced,
complex world.

As a chiropractor, people come to see me for a variety of
reasons including neck or back pain, headaches, digestion problems, depression, lowered states of energy or just a desire to be
healthier.

Like other holistic chiropractors, my first examination of a
new patient is far-reaching. First we collect detailed information to give us a picture of a patient's physical, mental and emotional state. Patients then describe their goals and expectations.
These might include decreased pain, more physical enjoyment
or a greater sense of well-being. Then together we form a treatment plan primarily designed to help empower that person's
innate healing abilities.

We perform a full analysis of the patient's spine and nervous
system including a posture assessment and physical exam. This
determines where tension and stress reside in the body and finds
any existing subluxation patterns. We do specialized testing of
the patient's autonomic, motor and sensory nervous systems
using a high-tech and high-touch approach.

We then guide the patient through a course of movements
and breathing. We do this while applying a series of gentle, precise contacts along the spine to areas called spinal gateways, which
are access points to the nervous system and areas where the vertebrae and spinal cord attach. The gentle, precise contacts help
the patient refocus on areas of spinal disturbance, creating more
understanding of what might be causing discomfort.

When patients become consciously and subconsciously more
aware of where they hold stress and tension in their bodies, they

can initiate self-correcting patterns or healing movements and learn how to properly release tensions.

Our work helps people become more aware of their bodies so their brains and nervous systems can find the problems. Simply put, in order to heal it, you have to first find it. When you can feel it, you can heal it.

For example, a patient may hold stress and tension in her neck. In times of "flight or fright" defense, her body's immediate reaction to trauma is to tense. Her muscles tightened, blood pressure rises and her emotions are subdued. Mental processing shifts from the highly-evolved, rational frontal cortex to more primitive, reactive areas of her brain. By contacting key points along her spinal cord in areas called "spinal gateways" with just the precise amount of force (often only ounces of pressure), in the precise direction and for the precise amount of time necessary, her nervous system's attention could be refocused towards healing and the generation of natural therapeutic movements. As her brain senses these contacts, it may become more aware of the spine, entire body and the connections within, thus unlocking the gateway to healing.

These gentle, precise contacts are called "entrainments" and essentially refocus and entrain the brain to learn new strategies for eliminating and dealing with stress, while greatly improving feelings of wellness.

In fact, NSA practitioners and neurobiologists theorize the subconscious portion of the brain is located in the spinal cord. This is actually neural tissue continuous with the brain. Releasing tension in the spinal cord could unlock the subconscious mind allowing it to go to work healing the body on an even deeper level. Through gentle and precise touch and breathing, the patient's mind is drawn to this area to help ease disproportionate tension, which could free the body to undertake a course of healing. As the spinal subluxations correct, these new strategies for deeper healing could be formed almost effortlessly.

The results could be astounding. By allowing the body to intelligently heal itself, you could experience fewer acute illnesses and possibly reduce chronic symptoms. Your energy levels could increase and overall physical well-being could improve. Many people report lower stress levels and better emotional states.

By reducing tension in the spinal cord, patients could learn to relax and may become more responsive to their emotional needs. This stress-free state may affect their lifestyle choices. Many of my patients, who become more conscious of the mind-body connection, start to exercise more, make better choices about foods and diets and improve their work and personal relationships. I believe they essentially get in touch with their "higher" selves and begin to listen to their inner voices more, which guide them towards healthier choices.

Doctors from the College of Medicine at the University of California conducted a research study with 2,818 patients who were under NSA care. The study concluded, "Results indicated that patients reported significant, positive perceived change in all four domains of health (physical, mental/emotional, stress evaluation and life enjoyment), as well as overall quality of life. The evidence of improved health suggests that Network Care (NSA) is associated with significant benefit. These benefits are evident from as early as one to three months under care and appear to show continuing clinical improvements in the duration of care intervals studied."

My patient, Courtney, age 28, had suffered for years from headaches, allergies and daily fatigue. During the gentle course of Network Care, Courtney experienced a new level of wellness. After just one week, the tension in her neck lessened. Her sleep became deeper. Now, she experiences fewer allergies, rarely has headaches and has the energy she had as a teenager. She feels more "in tune" with her body and is more able to fight off symptoms naturally when challenged by "what's going around." Her care has resulted in subsequent changes to her diet, her way of life, her relationships and her spiritual contentment.

I believe with NSA, the release of tension gives the brain an access point to the body, enabling it to find and analyze health problems. This tension release could also unleash energy trapped in tensed muscles and structures of the body. This energy could be applied as fuel for healing. So, the stress that could break us down could instead be energy that moves us toward wellness.

This gentle-touch chiropractic healing method could be used to unlock the mind-body connection of patients ranging from newborns to the elderly.

What is most wonderful is when children learn these healing strategies. They could learn to trust themselves more and how to release stress and tension effortlessly. My own daughter, Sophia, at age two, had been suffering from an ear infection. After just a few sessions not only had her ear infection cleared up, but her energy level also increased. Jordan, age six, had been a patient for only a few weeks when his mother remarked to us that all of her friends had told her that he has "really blossomed." He went from being a really shy and inward child to now being very sociable.

Another patient, Van, age 81, came to my office suffering from headaches and nearly constant pain and numbness. His medical doctors had encouraged surgery to relieve him from some of his discomfort. But after only a couple months of care, he experienced not only fewer and less frequent symptoms, but also rejuvenated energy. In fact, he has been so enthusiastic about learning more about health and well-being that he's attended several of my free lectures on wellness. He has embraced a new lifestyle of wellness for years to come. Each time he visits my office, I am deeply touched as he talks about the next five to ten years of increased health and vitality in his life.

Thomas Edison once said, "The doctor of the future will give no medicine but will interest the patient in the care of the human frame, and in the cause and prevention of disease." I believe the chiropractor is that "doctor of the future."

Chiropractors have been working with helping people regain their health for 109 years without recourse to drugs, surgery or risky, complicated interventions. We use only our hands, minds and hearts. Side effects, complications and malpractice suits are virtually unheard of with chiropractic care.

We believe the power that made the body heals the body when it is free from interference and is optimally focused. We believe a healthy nervous system naturally builds and rebuilds a fully healthy body. A healthy body nurtures and supports a healthy, flexible mind. Our primary goal is optimal health through optimal performance of the continuous web of nervous system tissue that includes the brain, spinal cord and the miles of sensory and motor nerves enlivening the entire body. We believe this system is the interface between the mind and the body and is the key to the health of the whole person.

A number of our patients say they enjoy freedom from pain, improved abilities to cope with stress, reduced fatigue, greater alertness and solid motivations toward healthier lifestyles. I have been blessed to witness many miracles like those of David, Vania, Van, Sophia and Courtney in my practice. By unlocking the mind-body connection, we could help patients become free from unnecessary pain, medications or surgeries and have personal experiences that they can trust their bodies more and embrace new lifestyles of wellness for years to come.

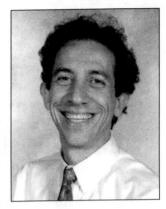

Elliott J. Mantell, D.C.
Common Ground Chiropractic
2927 NE Everett Street
Portland, Oregon 97232
(503) 232-4099
http://commonground.chiroweb.com
commonground@chiroenergy.com

Dr. Elliott J. Mantell, D.C., practices at Common Ground Wellness Center, a holistic healing center in Portland, Oregon. In 1973, he graduated from City University of New York. Then in 1980, he earned his Doctorate of Chiropractic degree from Western States Chiropractic College. While attending chiropractic college, he worked as a volunteer emergency medical technician (EMT). He started his private healing practice in 1981. Dr. Mantell is a member of the Association for Network Care and is certified in Network Spinal Analysis. He is also a member of the International Chiropractors Association (ICA), Waiting List Practice (WLP) and Parker Chiropractic Research Foundation (PCRF).

Dr. Mantell is constantly furthering his education to learn the most advanced techniques in chiropractic and natural healing methods throughout the United States and Europe.

For a complimentary consultation to see how Dr. Mantell's work could benefit you or to attend one of his many educational healing workshops, call his office at (503) 232-4099 or visit his web site at http://commonground.chiroweb.com .

PART EIGHT

NUTRITION BASED CHIROPRACTIC: THE FORGOTTEN FACTOR

Dr. Van D. Merkle, D.C., D.A.B.C.I., C.C.N.

If you are currently undergoing drug therapy for the treatment of a specific medical condition, are all the drugs you may be taking right now in your best interest?

The commonly prescribed antidepressant Prozac®, for example, can cause permanent nervous system damage, suicidal obsessions and acts of violence according to the recent report, *The Dangers of Prozac* by Dr. Gary Null, Ph.D. and Dr. Martin Feldman, M.D.

Even drugs as widely used and established as various allergy medications such as Allegra® can have side effects. According to Allegra's® official web site, side effects can include cold, flu, coughing, menstrual pain, sinusitis, backaches, accidental injury, insomnia, dizziness and nausea.

How many medications do you take a day? How many prescriptions do your parents take a day? For some people, the side effects of their pills could actually be more debilitating than the symptoms these drugs were originally prescribed to treat.

Individual Health

Nutrition Based Chiropractic has a remarkable tool that could make that goal of calculating individual health a reality.

Walk into most any chiropractic practice and you will likely meet a doctor who is willing to address nutritional issues, at least incidentally, by recommending a course of vitamins.

In my office, we do not rely on a one-size-fits-all vitamin. From our time with our patients, in addition to thorough examinations, we use surveys to gather comprehensive data to assess patients' health.

As a Chiropractic Internist and Nutritionist, I use a 52-point, comprehensive blood analysis that measures every leading health indicator from glucose levels to your specific white blood count. X-rays determine which areas of the spine need adjustment. A Nutrition Based Chiropractor relies on this bonanza of health information. This comes from blood, hair, urine and stool analysis. We use this information to determine exactly what sort of nutritional adjustments need to be made to help the particular individual achieve the best possible health.

I feel this type of metabolic and nutrition based practice has taken the guesswork out of chiropractic treatment. With laboratory testing, you receive real, measurable statistics presented in an easy-to-read numerical format. A patient's supplementation could be based on quantifiable facts presented by his or her individual blood chemistry.

As a patient's health improves, continued testing demonstrates how quickly health facts could change for the better. For most patients, seeing something like lower cholesterol numbers after only a few weeks of treatment provides all the incentive they'll need to stay on track.

Laboratory testing may sound like a radical departure from the ordinary, tried-and-true forms of chiropractic testing. Nutritional chiropractic practitioners do the exact same testing any other Doctor of Chiropractic might, like using X-rays and physical exams. He or she will still remove subluxations with spinal adjustments. The crucial difference lies in the fact Nutritional Based Chiropractic doesn't stop at adjusting the spine. Its practitioners treat the whole patient with the goal of searching out and reversing hidden conditions in blood levels before they become symptomatic or progress into dis-ease.

It's like stopping a forest fire at the first sign of smoke. With blood analysis, a Nutritional Based Chiropractor could detect and may end-run health challenges caused by improper nutrition. These conditions may include diabetes or high cholesterol.

By examining 52 separate serum profiles, the Nutrition Based Chiropractor could have the ability to bring the care of the entire body, and not just the spine, into healthy realignment. Environmental factors like chronic stress or impure drinking water are measured to determine the bearing they could have on blood levels of phosphorous or total protein.

I believe a healthy body doesn't ache. Also, I believe it is important to take all the side effects of drugs into account when deciding how to care for patients.

Many people turn to chiropractors as a last resort. These people might feel traditional medicine has failed them. If they don't get results from chiropractic care, they may feel doomed to suffer in accepting silence, frustrated and alone, with nowhere else to go.

Goal Of Nutrition Based Chiropractic

Nutrition Based Chiropractic was created with the goal of giving every patient a choice — particularly those patients who seem to have no other choice available.

If you are diagnosed with a disease, Nutrition Based Chiropractic could allow you to see your condition not as the disease alone, but as a series of chemical reactions, drug side effects and behaviors that could be affecting your entire body. Armed with this information, you could make adjustments to improve your health.

Once these adjustments are made, you could see improvement in your blood chemistry, your posture and even your lifestyle choices. This could bring your body back into balance and allow the body to heal naturally.

Today, with so many people taking multiple prescriptions and dealing with multiple side effects, it can be difficult to know which disorders are spontaneously appearing diseases and which are chemically self-induced. It is my belief that a full set of diagnostic tests on every patient, on a regular basis, is good practice. My desire is to take the focus off relieving symptoms and to look, instead, to the overall health of the human being.

If you are interested in taking advantage of Comprehensive Nutritional Blood Test Analysis, the test is available right now to every licensed chiropractor from coast-to-coast. Ask your chiropractor about the value of blood analysis. If you are a patient, ask your doctor to visit www.bk2health.com and ask about a test for you.

If you are a chiropractor, please stop by the website and learn how easy it is to offer this invaluable diagnostic tool to all your patients. You'll be amazed at how easy these reports are to read and understand.

Your body was created to be healthy. Give it the best environment possible and let it do what comes naturally.

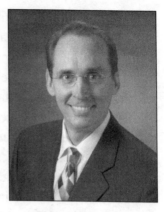

Dr. Van D. Merkle, D.C., D.A.B.C.I., C.C.N.
Back To Health Center
5761 Far Hills Avenue
Dayton, Ohio 45429
Phone (937) 433-3241
Fax (937) 439-0088
mail@bk2health.com
www.bk2health.com

Dr. Merkle is a Certified Clinical Nutritionist and a Doctor of Chiropractic. He has practiced in the Dayton, Ohio area for 18 years. A Diplomate on the American Chiropractic Board of Nutrition and a Diplomate on the American Board of Chiropractic Internists, he is also a member of The International and American Association of Clinical Nutritionists. Dr. Merkle has been host of the live, call-in talk show *Back To Health, Your Guide to Better Living* for over five years and frequently speaks to local groups and professionals around the country.

Located at 5761 Far Hills Ave in Dayton, Ohio, the Back To Health Center offers state-of-the-art diagnostic equipment and services to patients all over the United States. To schedule a private appointment with Dr. Merkle or to arrange for Dr. Merkle to speak to your corporation or group, call (937) 433-3241.

CHAPTER EIGHT

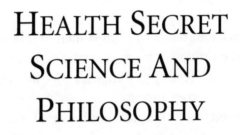

HEALTH SECRET
SCIENCE AND
PHILOSOPHY

PART ONE

WELLNESS STARTS HERE...

❧

Dr. Joseph Mannella, D.C.

Think back and recall your most memorable and fulfilling vacation. Take a moment to visualize the destination, the journey, the family or friends you were with. See the sights, sounds, and smells of the experience.

How did you feel on that vacation? Life was good, wasn't it?

Was that vacation a random act? Did it just happen out of the blue? Or did you PLAN and PREPARE FOR IT? Your vacation was a success because it not only met your expectations, it exceeded them! All of this is directly due to your planning and preparation of that destination.

Your health and wellness are also journeys that could have many different destinations. That destination *IS* your decision. I believe wellness starts the MOMENT you decide to plan it. The moment of any true decision changes your destiny. So to have wellness, one must first decide to achieve it. This may sound simple, but most people DON'T truly decide to achieve and sustain wellness. It's usually put off until you experience a crisis or significant health challenge.

Once you have decided to **BE** well, you must **DO** whatever it takes to **HAVE** wellness. **Be–Do–Have** is a great system for understanding the **achievement of wellness**. I believe wellness is achieved by BEING and DOING first. Then you could HAVE health and wellness. You can't skip the being and doing part and expect or demand the having part. It doesn't happen that way. Health and wealth are similar for the fact that you have to EARN both. True health and wellness cannot be bought. There is not a lottery for your health. It is up to YOU to decide if hoping or doing will take you to the health and wellness destination of your dreams.

I would like to congratulate you for having this book in your hands and continuing or starting your wellness journey. The most important part of any journey is the START. Know where you want to go. Learn everything you can to go in the right direction. Most importantly, take action and follow through because health and wellness come from you, not to you.

All success comes with a price. This is a combination of time, money and sacrifice. At every level of success, there will be an equal level of sacrifice. If you choose to be healthy for years to come, you will need to invest and sacrifice now. It seems counterintuitive to spend time and money or make a sacrifice when there isn't an immediate urgency, but that is the action necessary to propel your wellness intentions. Otherwise, you may be forced to spend your time and money fighting sickness and disease later. I'd rather be in control of my journey than end up in a place I never wanted to go.

Health And Wellness From The Beginning

Let us look back at how your health and wellness journey started. It actually started the moment you were conceived — one cell from dad and one cell from mom. Those two cells then combined into ONE CELL! Over time, that one cell started to divide and divide.

To control and coordinate your growth and connect you to this world, the brain, spinal cord and all the nerves of your body were the first tissues formed. Your brain, spinal cord and nerves were needed first! It is your antenna to the universe. It will process everything known and unknown for you to become you and to relate, coordinate and protect you in your environment. It started and sustains YOUR LIFE! That is why your spinal cord is often referred to as your "lifeline". This lifeline has a very real life force running over it from the time it was developed to this very moment and all the future moments of your life.

Please allow me to share with you my deep and spiritual view of health and wellness. Health comes from life. Life comes from God. God created the road to health and wellness first as your nervous system. I refer to it as a super highway. All functions and experiences exist because of this highway.

Don't search for new roads. Why not patch, repair and care for what God constructed for you? There will never be a single individual that could have the capacity to conceive of a different road.

God is in you, in all things, at all times. The God within us can flow normally or this power can be impeded. Bones out of place in your spine, called vertebral subluxations, could interfere with this God-given flow through your nerve system highway. Normal flow equals ease. Decreased flow equals dis-ease (not at ease). God never stops his flow from above down. Your subluxations could cause a loss or decrease of this never-ending flow from the inside out. Some drugs and medications could also decrease this natural flow. God will always be the source. You are responsible for maintaining the super highway. The way in which you maintain this super highway could affect your level of existence in relation to your God-given potential.

God directs man. Your nervous system directs YOU. I believe the God power within you is in your nervous system. Even if most people never learn this — that won't change this gift from God. Get to know the God WITHIN you seven days a week. Let it flow. Increase the flow and keep it flowing!

Respecting and caring for this incredible gift by proactively choosing health and wellness could be your greatest gift back to you and your Creator.

More To Health

Most people think they are achieving health and wellness if they simply exercise, eat a good diet and feel good in the moment. But, if your nervous system isn't functioning at 100 percent, can you truly be well? Being well isn't just how you feel. It's also how you function. Simply put, how you *are* is more important than how you *feel*.

That is why we need blood tests and nerve tests to tell us how we are before obvious symptoms and diseases develop. Symptoms are always the last to show up. They are the alarm; they are not the fire!

Doctors of Chiropractic specialize in detecting and correcting vertebral subluxations and nerve interference. The purpose of which is to allow your body to function at its highest level with ease. Doctors of Chiropractic give care and attention to spinal and nerve system health, which, in return, could help you achieve the true health and wellness you desire.

If an individual has a limiting belief about what creates health and wellness, they will be confined to that limiting belief's outcome. And unfortunately, they won't even see it coming. This book is great because it will cover things you know, things you don't know and, most importantly, things you aren't even aware that you didn't know. It's truly the things we don't know that we don't know that can hurt us the most.

Characteristics Of Successful Patients

What type of outcome will an individual with limited beliefs create? I'd like to see you expand the possibilities of what good health and wellness could look like for you.

Here are a few of the characteristics of my most successful wellness practice members:

1. They have an incredible **INTENTION** to get and stay well.
2. They believe life and health come from **above-down and inside-out.**

3. They are **decisive** and **take action**.
4. They are willing to **do and sacrifice** whatever it takes to win this game.
5. They make their **own decisions** about their modes of healthcare.
6. **They love doing what they believe is right for them!**
7. They understand wellness is about the **journey**.
8. They **persist** with what they have started.
9. They **learn from their mistakes.**
10. They know **success leaves clues.**

I hope your wellness path continues and broadens as you increase your personal appreciation of yourself, your nervous system and your freedom of healthcare choices.

Share this information with everyone you know to give them the opportunities of true wellness. This world can absolutely be a better place when all are well.

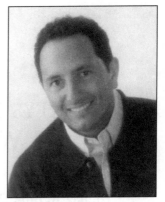

Dr. Joseph Mannella, D.C.
Family Chiropractic
67421 Main Street
Richmond, Michigan 48062
Phone: (586) 727-7557
Fax (586) 727-6441
www.drmannella.com
drjoe@drmannella.com

In addition to an active family practice, Dr. Mannella is the inventor of a posture correcting orthopedic device called the Posture Right™ Neck Orthotic for neck, head, TMJ and posture problems. This device is helping thousands of people correct a very common, but extremely serious condition called forward head posture. For more information on the Posture Right™ Neck Orthotic, go to www.postureright.com or call (586) 727-7557.

By age 11, Dr. Joseph Mannella made a genuine decision to become a Doctor of Chiropractic. At age 23, Dr. Mannella opened his first office and has opened a total of seven successful practices to date.

Dr. Mannella consulted for one of the largest chiropractic consulting firms and traveled extensively giving his own seminars to health professionals.

With drugs and surgery increasing, Dr. Mannella realized the chiropratic truth and wellness principles were being missed by many.

His deep passion for sharing wellness principles and witnessing miracles through chiropractic keeps him going and appreciating the opportunity God has given him to serve.

If you would like to schedule a private appointment with Dr. Mannella or would like him to speak to your corporation or group, call (586) 727-7557.

PART TWO

SIX KEYS TO HEALTH AND WELLNESS

✎

Dr. Joel W. Bird, D.C., IDE, QME, CCST, MUAC

Is health and wellness the absence of disease? Is it "not feeling bad?" Is it just having a great day?

Throughout my research, I have found the most logical and complete definition of health and wellness is comprised of six keys:

1. Structural integrity of the musculoskeletal/nervous system;
2. Removal of extra exposure to electrical pollution;
3. Emotional stability;
4. Absence of nutritional deficiency;
5. Decreasing sensitivity to allergies; and
6. Decreasing toxicity levels in the body.

If all the keys are not present, in my opinion, health and wellness remain elusive and locked away.

According to findings by The Institute for Organ Transplantation and Immunocytology in Italy as reported by Pubmed.com in an article referenced on the site as PMID14603534: "It has been recently established that low-frequency electromagnetic field exposure induces biological changes and could be associated with increased incidence of cancer."

Fifty hour work weeks, marital problems, traffic, pollution, our increasing dependence on electricity and decreasing nutritional value in our foods are only a few of the things in our lives that make the goal of health and wellness a modern day struggle.

I believe wellness is not just "feeling okay" or the absence of disease. So, how do we achieve health and wellness in our current lives?

The foundation of health is in the structural integrity of the musculoskeletal and nervous systems. All tissues in the body need nerve function. If the nerves are not functioning properly, neither will the tissues supplied by those nerves. If tissues, muscles or connective tissue are restricted, this could decrease the functional integrity of the nervous system. Decreasing the functional capacity of the nervous system could be extremely detrimental to overall health and wellness.

As much as we don't want to believe this, research has shown overexposure to electrical waves and electromagnetic energy could block our ability to achieve health and wellness. It is my opinion, the frequency of metabolic diseases, autoimmune diseases, childhood illnesses, psychiatric diseases and many other conditions seem to correlate with our increased dependence on electricity.

Our homes and offices are full of machines using alternating current (AC). This may be known to interfere with the human nervous system, which is direct current (DC).

If you don't believe bodies are electromagnetic in nature then why, when you jump in the air, don't you stay in the air? That is because the earth has a magnetic core, which creates gravity. Gravity is a magnetic force that pulls our electromagnetic bodies toward the earth.

Nutritional deficiencies in our daily diet are a major problem in our industrialized society. How many fast food restaurants can you name? In our busy lives, fast food has become the rule when, I believe, it really should be an exception.

There are water sources polluted with polychlorinated biphenals (PCBs), arsenic and mercury where fish and other seafood we eat become contaminated. Our Federal government has recently produced guidelines stating pregnant women and children should limit their intakes of tuna or other types of seafood since mercury content can harm developing nervous systems. Our fruits and vegetables are watered and grown with this same polluted water.

The food we eat every day may be full of ingredients that preserve our food, but doesn't preserve our health and wellness.

Our organs, glands, musculoskeletal system and nervous system must function optimally to maintain our health and wellness. These systems require proper nutrition. Proper nutrition for our organ systems means the presence of the proper enzymes and/ or acid levels to promote proper digestion of foods, assimilation of nutrients and elimination of wastes.

Emotional Beings

Some might say emotions do not play a part in the status of your health and wellness. However, research and books have shown emotions are a cornerstone for health and wellness. It is becoming clear how emotions correlate with the state of a person's health.

This emotion based body-mind correlation results in chemical reactions in the brain, tissue and cells, which produce energy. This energy can be either positive or negative. Researcher Candice Pert Ph.D. states in her book, *Molecules of Emotion*, all emotions, both negative and positive, are healthy emotions. It is when we repress these emotions and don't let them flow freely that we create a dis-integrity in the system. This causes the body to not work as a unified whole.

Dr. Pert states stress could create weakened conditions within our bodies which might lead to disease. Health and wellness is more than just thinking happy thoughts. It is the realization all *honest* emotions are *positive* emotions when expressed and not hidden.

Toxins are prevalent in our current surroundings. Toxic metals are used in various industries and a number of these heavy metals find their way into our food, air and water. When these toxins accumulate in our tissues and cells, they could cause cellular mutation or cellular death. When a person is exposed to various toxins, he or she might suffer from headaches, fatigue, skin disorders, asthma, allergies and muscle and joint pain. Some of these toxins might affect the brain and could create challenges with memory, thought processes and even moods.

Your Doctor of Chiropractic who is trained in wellnesscare can test for most of the interferences affecting health and wellness. When interference is identified, your Doctor of Chiropractic can help you eliminate, control, give nutritional supplementation for and stabilize interferences so the body can express its homeostasis.

As defined in *Mosby's Medical Dictionary 4ᵗʰ Edition*, "homeostasis is a relative constancy in the internal environment of the body, naturally maintained by adaptive response, which promotes healthy survival. Some of the key control mechanisms are the reticular formation in the brainstem and the endocrine glands. Some of the functions controlled by homeostatic mechanisms are the heartbeat, hematopoiesis (the normal function and development of blood cells), blood pressure, body temperature, electrolytic balance, respiration and glandular secretion."

Simply stated, homeostasis is the ability or tendency of an organism or cell to maintain equilibrium by adjusting its physiological processes.

If you have any of the six major interferences, mentioned previously, you cannot achieve homeostasis.

I feel health and wellness are journeys — not destinations. We are bombarded with the interferences mentioned. It is my belief we must be continually monitored for such interference and cared for accordingly.

As a Doctor of Chiropractic, I believe people need to be evaluated for such interferences and treated honestly, ethically and correctly. With appropriate chiropractic care, nutritional evaluation and emotional stabilization, we could all achieve homeostasis, health and overall wellness.

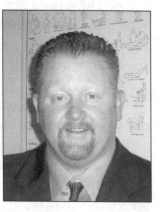

Dr. Joel W. Bird, D.C., IDE, QME, CCST, MUAC
Advanced Wellness & Chiropractic
2276 South Figueroa Street
Los Angeles, California 90007
Phone (213) 747-4287
Fax (213) 747-4387
www.DrJoelBird.com

Dr. Joel W. Bird, D.C. is a practicing Doctor of Chiropractic, an industrial disability examiner and a qualified medical examiner. Dr. Bird holds certificates in chiropractic spinal trauma and manipulation under anesthesia. Dr. Bird has also published research in the *Journal of Manipulative and Physiologic Therapeutics* and is currently furthering his research and understanding into health and wellness.

Information regarding the FDA and its opinions regarding nutrition can be viewed at www.cfsan.fda.gov .

To schedule a private appointment with Dr. Bird or to arrange for Dr. Bird to speak to your corporation or group, call (213) 747-4287.

PART THREE

BUILDING BLOCKS OF LIFE

Dr. John Jung, D.C., FIAMA

Amino acids are building blocks of protein and hormones. I believe the benefits of amino acids are underestimated. Chiropractors are well educated in the field of nutrition and are able to help in providing information on amino acids.

Digestive enzymes and water break down proteins into amino acids, which are absorbed and transported by the blood to various body tissues. The body uses amino acids for repair, maintenance and growth.

Some amino acids can be created by the body. These are called non-essential amino acids. Others must be included in the diet and are known as essential amino acids.

Here is a list of some of the amino acids we work with at our clinic:

Alanine

Alanine can be created within the body. This amino acid could help in the stabilization of blood sugar levels. Along with other amino acids, alanine may play a role in supporting prostate health. Some protein-rich plant foods supply alanine along with meat, eggs, poultry, fish and dairy.

Arginine

Arginine can be created within the body. The pituitary gland requires this amino acid, along with others, for proper release of growth hormones. It can assist in wound healing and stimulating immune function.

Aspartic acid

Aspartic acid can be created within the body. Its purpose is to assist the body in ridding toxic ammonia and helping to protect the central nervous system.

Cysteine and Cystine

The body converts cystine into cysteine as needed. When this happens, it creates a substance which helps detoxify the body. Cysteine may help strengthen the stomach and intestine lining. It may also help communication within the immune system.

N-acetyl Cysteine

As a precursor to glutathione, I have used this for alcoholics, hangovers and analgesic abuse. The antioxidant activity may act as a buffer against free radicals.

Glutamic acid

The brain uses glutamic acid to help remove surplus ammonia. Glutamate is a stimulating neurotransmitter in the central nervous system. Glutamic acid is found in prostate fluid and may play a role in the normal function of the prostate. Glutamic acid may also help the heart muscle. Sources include poultry, meat, fish, eggs and dairy.

Glutamine

Glutamine is found in plant and animal proteins. It is also created by the body. Glutamine has been shown to help control sugar cravings because the body can convert it to glucose. It is also important for immune function. It is found in high protein foods such as meat, beans, fish and dairy.

Glycine

Glycine is produced by the body. The body uses glycine to build proteins. It is also known to help the brain's chemical messengers involved in memory. Glycine can be found in high protein foods such as meat, dairy, fish and beans.

Histidine

This is known as a semi-essential amino acid. Why? Adults may produce enough, but children may not. Histidine is a predecessor to histamine, which is released by the immune system to fight allergic reactions. Sources are dairy, meat, fish and poultry.

Lysine

This essential amino acid is not produced by the body, which means it must be supplied by diet or supplements. Lysine is important to proteins used by the body. Research has shown lysine hinders the growth of certain herpes viruses. In addition to supplements, lysine can be found in Brewer's yeast, dairy, fish, meat and legumes.

Methionine

Methionine cannot be produced by the body. Therefore, it must be provided in the diet or by supplementation. Methionine helps metabolism and growth. It belongs to a group of compounds called lipotropics (lipids) that helps the liver process fat. Research suggests people with AIDS have lower levels of methionine.

Good sources of methionine include fish, dairy, meat and whole grains.

Phenylalanine and DL-Phenylalanine (DLPA)

Phenylalanine is an essential amino acid that helps communication between nerve cells and the brain. This group includes DL-phenylalanine, DLPA, DPA, LPA and L-phenylalanine. Certain members of this group appear to work with brain chemicals relating to pain sensation and mood elevation.

L-Tyrosine

The body creates tyrosine from another amino acid called phylalanine. Tyrosine has a role in brain activity. It is also converted into melanin by the skin cells. This is the dark pigment used by the body to protect against harm from ultraviolet rays. Tyrosine can be found in thyroid hormones and in protein-rich foods such as dairy, meat, fish and wheat.

At the forefront of nutrition breakthroughs today, enzymes and amino acid supplementation are providing innovative methods to help the body's performance. While nutrition is part of the overall body's function (and in certain circumstances amino acids may have therapeutic effects) this does not make enzymes and amino acids universally applicable in all named conditions since no single nutrient can resolve all such cases.

The correct use of any nutrient in any health problem is to provide the body with what it needs on a biochemical level. We must further research the interactions of nutrients with each other to employ safe and effective therapies.

Call or write my office for a complete listing of dosages specific for your health concern.

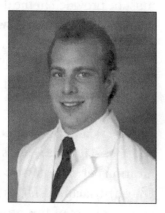

Dr. John Jung, D.C., FIAMA
1506 Arlington Heights Road
Arlington Heights, Illinois 60004
(847) 255-3443

Dr. John Jung received high honors from the American Holistic College of Nutrition, Diplomate of International Academy of Acupuncture, BA degree from Illinois Weslyan University, B.S. degree from National College of Chiropractic, certified in Manipulation Under Anesthesia. Dr. Jung's practice is 50 percent internal medicine.

To schedule a private appointment with Dr. Jung or to arrange for Dr. Jung to speak to your corporation or group, call (847) 255-3443.

CHAPTER NINE

WHIPLASH AND INJURY HEALTH SECRET

PART ONE

What You Must Know
If You Have Been
In An Accident

∽

Dr. Michael Brady, D.C., F.A.S.A

Wellness is your greatest asset. I have been helping people achieve wellness through chiropractic for nearly two decades.

What is wellness? Wellness is when all cells, tissues and organs are working at optimal levels 100 percent of the time. Wellness is truly an inside job.

I believe wellness is best achieved when the central nervous system, comprised of the brain and spinal cord, are free of nerve interference. The central nervous system is the communication control center of the body.

Electrically Operating

Electrical signals are generated by the brain. They travel from the brain through nerves, up and down the spinal cord where they branch out to various parts of your body.

Chiropractic care could help the central nervous system work properly by relieving pressure on nerves caused by spinal misalignments or subluxations.

With a properly functioning central nervous system, the body may be able to increase its healing abilities.

Despite our best efforts to maintain wellness, forces outside our control can disrupt it. For instance, an automobile accident can be very traumatic for the human body and cause a variety of injuries from broken bones to serious soft tissue damage.

Most of the injuries I treat are to soft tissue. You don't have to have broken bones to have significant disabilities.

A typical rear-end collision puts a tremendous amount of stress on the spine — particularly the neck. While a seat belt holds your torso and pelvis in place, it doesn't do anything to support your neck. It's important to understand even low speed automobile accidents can be very damaging to the body.

The human head weighs about as much as a bowling ball. A rear-end collision can place significant force on the neck, even if for a split second.

When spinal misalignment occurs as a result of a rear-end accident, overall wellness can be disrupted. Symptoms may include neck and back pain, muscle spasms, loss of strength, decreased range of motion, headaches, nervousness, the inability to sleep and numbness and/or tingling in the arms and legs.

A patient of mine was involved in a motor vehicle accident. She was stopped when her vehicle was hit hard from behind. She immediately started having severe neck and back pain. She started to get a terrible headache that radiated from her neck up the back of her head to her eye. She knew she was in trouble. She was taken to the hospital where she was X-rayed and given a muscle relaxant and a painkiller. However, she felt the only way to get back to true wellness was to see me for an examination and to establish a treatment plan.

She couldn't move her head. She had no strength in her left arm. She felt miserable.

Upon examination, I found she had swelling in her neck. She couldn't move her head because of vertebral subluxation. The impact from the accident forced her cervical vertebrae out of proper alignment, stretched muscles and tore ligaments in her neck. This vertebral misalignment in her lower neck placed pressure on the nerves running down her left arm.

I performed a surface electromyogram (SEMG). This is a computerized test that reveals the amount of electrical activity in the muscles. The test confirmed she had significant muscle spasms.

I also performed strength testing that revealed a loss of strength in her left upper extremity. Careful palpation (examination by hand) revealed a bump or nodule on the left side, midway down her neck.

I used ice packs to reduce the swelling. After several chiropractic adjustments, her symptoms started to improve. The swelling in her neck was gone. Her range of motion improved. The patient could turn her head again and was able to return to work.

X-rays revealed she had lost the normal curve in her neck. Her neck was curving the wrong way from the torn ligaments. I showed her the results of her tests. I explained that once she was out of pain, we would need to restore her normal cervical curve to fully regain proper function of her spine and nervous system.

She followed my instructions and did her exercises. After a few months, she was back to normal. After her full recovery, she was ready for wellnesscare. She continues to exercise, eat smart and receives chiropractic care to maintain her health.

I feel that with proper chiropractic care, she was able to avoid a dangerous surgery on her neck.

Many people associate whiplash injury with automobile accidents. However, a whiplash-type injury doesn't only occur in automobile accidents. Whiplash injuries may occur as a result of sudden forces to the body from such contact sports as football or soccer. Whiplash-type injuries can occur with falls or direct traumas to the skull. Even a sudden sneeze can cause whiplash.

Following a whiplash injury, there may be neck soreness and stiffness as the muscles contract in their attempts to pull the head and spine back into alignment. I believe anyone sustaining a minor whiplash injury should have his or her spine checked.

Treating a spinal misalignment with the goal of achieving wellness involves a step-by-step plan to be followed by the patient and the chiropractor.

In my practice, patients first undergo comprehensive orthopedic and neurological spinal exams. Some may require an MRI or CT scan, if clinically indicated.

After the exam, I review all examination findings from the diagnostic procedures. I develop treatment plans that help patients regain their health. Such a plan may consist of gentle spinal manipulation to correct the subluxations.

I construct a care plan tailor-made for the needs of each particular patient. Some care plans may be short in duration and some may be longer.

Regardless of the length of the plan, I believe wellness is achieved when the nervous system is functioning properly. The central nervous system is the main communication system within the body. I feel if the nervous system is not functioning properly, we can never truly be healthy. I show my patients how chiropractic care and adjustments can remove subluxations and nerve interference that could help the body heal itself.

Regardless of the reason for the initial visit, I hope patients view chiropractic care in a different light after their first adjustment.

Upon realizing the wonderful benefits of chiropractic care, a number of patients choose to become lifetime, wellnesscare patients. These patients come in periodically to enhance their well-being and feel better, not just when they are in pain.

I believe that, like professional athletes, patients who receive periodic chiropractic care stay closer to optimal performance. I believe they look better, have increased immune systems and have more energy.

Now, you too could enjoy the most out of life while feeling your best!

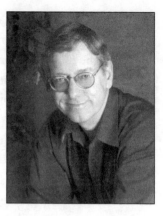

Dr. Michael Brady, D.C., F.A.S.A
Accident and Injury Center
1232 NW Harrison Street
Topeka, Kansas
(785) 232-9900
www.DrMikeBrady.TopChiro.com

Dr. Brady is a native of Topeka, Kansas. He has helped thousands of people regain their health through natural methods. Dr. Brady is a leading authority who has appeared on radio and television. He regularly lectures on healthcare and back and neck injuries.

Dr. Brady graduated from Cleveland Chiropractic College with postgraduate studies in orthopedics and specialized training in pain management. Dr. Brady has over 45,000 hours of clinical experience.

Dr. Brady is certified in physiotherapy from Cleveland Chiropractic College. He is nationally and internationally certified in Clinical Acupuncture. He holds post-graduate certification in Impairment and Disability ratings, Applied Spinal Disability and a master certification in Performance of AMA Permanent Medical Impairment Examinations.

Dr. Brady is a member of the Kansas Chiropractic Foundation, Fellow of Acupuncture Society of America, Diplomat of the American Academy of Pain Management, Affiliate Member of the Medical Legal Consultants Association and Certified Member of the North American Academy of Impairment Rating Physicians. He has been featured in *National Who's Who* Directory of Executives and Professionals and *Oxford's Who's Who* Elite Registry of Extraordinary Professionals.

For a private appointment with Dr. Brady or to schedule Dr. Brady to speak for your corporation or group, call (785) 232-9900.

PART TWO

"Whiplash"
An American Epidemic

❧

Dr. Gary Anglen, D.C.

I have over 18 years of experience treating whiplash victims. One thing is clear — there are a number of myths and misunderstandings about whiplash. Millions of Americans suffer the pains of whiplash.

The neck injury that occurs with whiplash trauma is complex and highly variable. This is due to the wide range of occupants' physical make-ups and postures along with pre-collision conditions. However, an injury model has been developed which generally describes the whiplash trauma which could occur from rear impact collisions.

One of the harshest forces on the human body is in rear impact trauma. Forces such as this are rarely seen elsewhere. These forces are horizontal shear forces. They are experienced while the neck is compressed. The compression loosens ligaments increasing joint play and joint injuries. The second factor is the extreme short timing of the accident. Injuries could occur within 100th to 125th of a millisecond.

Having participated in live crash testing, it was shocking the first time I saw a low speed collision. The car was traveling so slowly. Yet the noise upon impact was so loud. Even with a trained eye and understanding of what was happening, the collision was over in a flash.

I have asked patients about their crashes. Many have responded saying, "It was so violent! I was shocked! But my head did not move! All I know was that it was loud! I don't want to go through it again!"

When I have shown patients a human volunteer crash film, some gasp in disbelief. An occasional patient says, "That is not what happened to me. I hardly moved."

Yet they were in my office with neck pains and stiffness.

Class Of Its Own

Whiplash injuries have been compared by some to sports traumas. Sports injures are significantly different. The mechanism of whiplash is unique. It should not be related to sports trauma or other self-induced injures.

Primarily, the extremely short duration and the formation of the unstable S-curve in the neck are two keys explaining why rear impacts have significantly higher injury rates.

Long-term pain and spinal instabilities could be the result of stretched joint capsules, pinched discs and other joints, stretched vertebral arteries and intersegmental hyperextension at lower cervical levels. Spinal instabilities could be due to compromised ligamentous subfailure, the tearing of small joints of the spine and disc injuries.

These injuries may not be detected on plain X-rays or MRIs. However, they could be evaluated, to a degree, with stress radiographs, templating and digitization. To evaluate the quality of motion during movement when joint laxities are suspected, I feel digital motion fluoroscopy is the best diagnostic tool available.

Autopsies of whiplash victims who have died from other means, show a variety of whiplash complications ranging from pulled muscles to brain stem injuries.

Nerve injuries could occur when nerves are stretched and torn even while protective sheaths are still intact.

I believe whiplash is an American epidemic.

According to a review by Dr. Michael Freeman, Dr. Arthur Croft and others published in *Spine*, Volume 42, Number 1, page

86-98, "The National Highway Traffic Safety Administration reports that, in 1995 there were 5,500,000 Americans injured in motor vehicle crashes. A large, population-based study found that 53 percent of injuries include whiplash injuries, amounting to 2,900,000 acute whiplash cases in 1995."

The report goes on to say of those suffering whiplash, 33 percent of whiplash victims still suffered the injury at 33 months. The authors estimated for 1995 as many as 90,000 people suffered the symptoms and effects of whiplash for the first time several months after the actual injuries were sustained.

The authors go on to conservatively calculate that 6.2 percent of the American population or 15,500,000 Americans have late whiplash.

Whiplash victims could continue to be symptomatic for years after the injury. Studies show neck pain, headaches and arm pain are among the most debilitating symptoms.

Whiplash symptoms do not always start at the scene of the accident. The first stage of healing could take 72 hours and swelling could continue for days. Whiplash symptoms could appear several months later.

In an unlikely twist of irony, it was orthopedic surgeons Martin Gargan and Gordon Bannister who joined forces with a chiropractor and published the first study supporting chiropractic care in the treatment of late whiplash. In the study of late whiplash it was reported that 26 of 28 chiropractic patients or 93 percent found improvement in chronic symptoms. Another of their studies resulted in 69 of 93 patients improving following chiropractic care.

"Whiplash injuries are common. Chiropractic is the only proven effective treatment in chronic cases," according to the conclusion of a study by the University Department of Orthopaedic Surgery, Bristol, United Kingdom entitled *A Symptomatic Classification of Whiplash Injury and the Implications for Treatment* by Khan, Cook, Gargan and Bannister published in *The Journal of Orthopaedic Medicine* 21(1) 1999.

Higher Speeds

Crash testing has revealed new information about most modern passenger vehicles. A number of modern vehicles can withstand crash speeds of up to 8 to 10 mph — and often higher — without sustaining visible damage.

According to a study by Malcolm Robbins entitled *Lack of Relationship Between Vehicle Damage and Occupant Injury*, it states, "A common misconception formulated is that the amount of vehicle crash damage due to a collision offers a direct correlation to the degree of occupant injury."

His study further states, "This false reasoning often applied by insurance adjusters, attorneys and physicians…the injured parties often are not compensated, resulting in unjustified hardship to the party who has already been injured."

The conclusion made by some is that when little or no vehicle body or bumper damage occurs, even though vehicles may be subject to fairly serious collisions, there is no occupant injury. The flaw in this conclusion is that solid bumper-to-bumper chassis can sustain higher impacts and show little or no damage. Yet, the occupants' bodies are not made of bumper-to-bumper, high grade metal and can, therefore, sustain severe injuries while the vehicle sustains little or no damage. Crash damage does not relate to occupant injury.

Some experts reported the threshold for soft tissue injury of the neck — in healthy adult males in proper body positions and aware of the impending impact — may happen at vehicle speed changes of only 5 mph. However, modern passenger vehicles can crash at nearly twice this injury threshold, yet appear undamaged. New crash tests indicate that a change of vehicle velocity of only 2.5 mph may produce occupant injuries in real world occupants.

New scientific studies from Japan conclude there is a lack of relationship between occupant injury, vehicle speed and damage. There does not seem to be an absolute speed or amount of damage a vehicle sustains in order for a person to experience injury.

Probably the most important thing for a doctor to evaluate,

in addition to the patient, is the risk factors of the occupant in the crash. There are specific risk factors that have been reported in the literature about acute and late whiplash.

I would like to share a short story with you about a patient named Richard. He was in an accident over 14 years ago. He was a truck driver driving from Redding to Reno on Highway 299 east bound. This was a trip he had probably made a hundred times before. He was rounding a curve when he saw a station wagon filled with people turned across the road. Richard knew if he hit it, all those people would be killed. He quickly turned his diesel into the embankment. As he was braking, the truck skidded sideways. He was able to keep it from flipping over onto the station wagon by steering it off the road. The truck went off the road and down a steep hillside where he hit a large pine tree.

Richard's body was thrown across the cab of the truck where he hit the metal door. The impact of his body made an indentation in the door.

Richard was transported by emergency medical services to the hospital. He was in intensive care for days and in the hospital for weeks. He underwent many tests. His medical doctor treated him with drugs, physiotherapy and rehabilitation.

Richard suffered broken bones, herniated discs, torn nerves and pulled muscles and ligaments. Richard was unable to return to work for about ten years. He was referred to me. I think Richard said it best, "Chiropractic is about quality of life. When I'm treated, I feel better and the pain is manageable."

An informed patient understands the goals of their treatment. Realistic expectations of treatment outcomes increase a patient's satisfaction.

Injuries Present Themselves Over Time

The sad thing is when whiplash victims do not understand the significant injury which could occur due to whiplash traumas. They prematurely dismiss whiplash based on an absence of pain without addressing potentially injured tissues. This could be setting the stage for chronic problems to occur as joint degeneration may follow in the decades to come.

One of the most insidious symptoms is a headache which may start years after the trauma due to the build up of muscle tension. Some patients with significant chronic pain from whiplash injuries could, over time, develop cognitive dysfunction, emotional changes and depression.

Chiropractic Has Stood Test Of Time

Chiropractic manipulation has passed the test of time. It was practiced by ancient Chinese, Hindu, Mayan, Aztec, Egyptian and numerous other peoples throughout history. Methodical scientific studies have validated chiropractic manipulation for the treatment of whiplash injuries.

Patients think it's a miracle when their pains go away. In my opinion, the miracle is God has given us such an easy way to positively affect the nervous system.

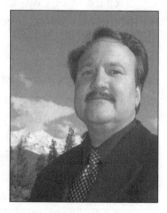

Dr. Gary Anglen, D.C.
Health Quest Chiropractic
465 Lake Boulevard
Redding, California
(530) 243-8157
www.doctor-anglen.com

Dr. Anglen has post-graduate studies in spinal trauma, whiplash injuries and accident reconstruction. He has participated in human volunteer accident crash testing. He is an active member of Center for Research into Automotive Safety and Heath (CRASH), Association for the Advancement of Automotive Medicine (AAAM), Society of Automotive Engineers (SAE), Council on Applied Chiropractic Science (CACS), California Chiropractic Association (CCA) and National Association for Seatbelt Safety Awareness (NASSA). Dr. Anglen has earned Chiropractic Certification in Spinal Trauma (CCST) as presented by the International Chiropractors Association and certification in collision reconstruction as presented by Texas A&M.

To schedule a private appointment with Dr. Anglen or arrange for him to speak to your corporation or group, call (530) 243-8157.